THE EMOTION CODE

**How to Release Your Trapped Emotions
for Abundant Health, Love and Happiness**

THE EMOTION CODE

**How to Release Your Trapped Emotions
for Abundant Health, Love and Happiness**

Dr. Bradley Nelson

Wellness Unmasked Publishing
Mesquite, Nevada

First Edition, June 2007

Published in the United States by Wellness Unmasked Publishing,
a division of Wellness Unmasked Incorporated, Mesquite, Nevada.
"The Emotion Code", "Heart-Wall", and "Body Code"
are trademarks of Wellness Unmasked, Inc.

Library of Congress Control Number: 2007928684
Nelson, B. (Bradley), 1957-
The Emotion Code: How to Release Your Trapped Emotions
for Abundant Health, Love and Happiness / Dr. Bradley Nelson.
p. cm.
Includes bibliographic references and index.
ISBN 978-0-9795537-0-7 (pbk.)

Printed in the United States of America

DEDICATION

To the memory of Bruce A. Nelson, Sr. and Ruth Nelson, my wonderful parents, who always loved and believed in me. My only regret is not finishing this book while they were yet alive, but I feel sure they have seen it anyway.

To the memory of Doctors Ida Glynn Harmon and Allen Baine, (Doc and Ida) who healed my body when I was a very sick boy and introduced me to the world of natural healing.

To Dr. Stanley Flagg, my teacher and mentor.

Finally, to my wife Jean, whose ideas, insights, contributions, dreams and support made this work possible.

A NOTE TO READERS

The Emotion Code is a self-help method that quite often produces marvelous results and wonderful benefits, both physical and emotional in nature. Nevertheless, it is a relatively new discovery and has not been thoroughly studied.

This book is based on the personal observations and experiences of Dr. Bradley Nelson. You, the reader, must take 100% responsibility for your own health, both physical and emotional. The Emotion Code should not be misconstrued or used to diagnose the presence or absence of any particular mental, physical or emotional ailment. Neither muscle testing nor the Sway Test should be used to diagnose the presence or absence of disease.

This book is not intended to be a substitute for the services of any health care professional. Neither the author nor the publisher is responsible for any consequences incurred by those employing the remedies or treatments discussed or taught herein. Any application of the material set forth in the following pages is at the reader's discretion and is his or her sole responsibility. The information contained in these materials is intended for personal use and not for the practice of any healing art, except where permitted by law. No representation contained in these materials is intended as medical advice and should not be used for diagnosis or medical treatment.

The stories in this book are all true, but the names have been changed in some circumstances to protect privacy.

CONTENTS

PART IV A BRIGHTER FUTURE

The Refiner's Fire of Life —357
About Prayer—359

ACKNOWLEDGEMENTS

My express thanks go out to those who have helped in the creation of this work.

To my patients, for allowing me to be their friend and doctor, and for allowing me to share their stories.

To my brother Greg, for introducing me to magnetic healing and to a new way of seeing things.

To my brother Bruce, for teaching me about the power of intention and the power of charity.

To my sisters Michele and Noelle, for their positive encouragement and love.

To Donna Beech for listening to me for hours on end, and for organizing my material and helping me to get started.

To Jean and Natalie Nelson and Ryan Muirhead for their excellent help with editing and photography.

To Kristi, Natalie, Jean, Rhett, Ian, Elisabeth, Angela, Noelle and Cierra for modeling, and to Drew and Joseph for their ideas and positive input.

To Joseph, for his artistic input and creativity, and to Drew for being so supportive and helpful.

To Isamu Masuda, for his dream of healing the world and for creating the magnetic tools to do just that.

To my wife Jean, for sticking with me through thick and thin, for being my inspiration, my helper and my best friend.

Finally, to God for answering my prayers, for blessing me with the gifts I would need to accomplish this work, for making me an instrument of healing, and for guiding my life all along the way.

PART I

TRAPPED EMOTIONS

TRUTH IS STRANGER THAN FICTION, BUT THIS IS
BECAUSE FICTION IS OBLIGED TO STICK TO PROBABILITY;
TRUTH IS NOT.

- MARK TWAIN

1

TRAPPED EMOTIONS:
THE INVISIBLE EPIDEMIC

Where would you be without your emotions? If the sum total of all your experiences makes up the tapestry of your life, it is the emotions you have experienced that give that tapestry its color.

Our emotions really do give color to our lives. Try to imagine for a moment a world where no emotions could occur. No joy would be possible. No feelings of happiness, bliss, charity or kindness. No love would be felt, no positive emotions of any kind.

On this imaginary emotionless planet, there would be no negative emotions either. No sorrow, no anger, no feelings of depression, and no grief. To live on such a planet would be to merely exist. With no ability to feel emotions of any kind, life would be reduced to a gray, mechanical ritual from cradle to grave. Be grateful that you can feel emotions!

But are there emotions you have experienced that you would rather not have felt? If you are like most people, your life has had its darker times. You have probably experienced moments of anxiety, as well as other times of grief, anger, frustration, and fear. You may have experienced periods of sorrow, as well as depression, low self-esteem, hopelessness, or any of a wide variety of negative emotions.

What you may not realize is that some of the negative emotions you've experienced, even though you may have felt them long ago, may still be creating problems for you in subtle, yet very damaging ways. The Emotion Code is about finding those old emotions and releasing them forever.

Much of our suffering is due to negative emotional energies that have become 'trapped' within us. The Emotion Code is a simple and powerful method of finding and releasing these trapped energies.

Many people have found that when they free themselves of their trapped emotions they are able to live healthier and happier lives. A single trapped emotion can create both physical and emotional problems.

The following real-life examples illustrate how releasing trapped emotional energy using the Emotion Code can result in astonishing and sudden improvements in physical and emotional wellness:

Allison's debilitating hip pain left her instantly, and she was able to dance in her performance that night...

Linda's constant feelings of suicidal depression went away...

Jennifer's chronic anxiety was gone, and she now felt the total confidence she'd been longing for...

Laurie reported that for the first time in her life, she could feel God's love for her...

Sheryl was finally able to shed her anger for her ex-husband, and create a wonderful, loving relationship with a new man...

Julia aced her court reporting test, after failing several times...

Larry's foot pain disappeared along with his limp...

Connie's allergies disappeared...

Neil's 2 year-long feeling of resentment for his boss vanished...

Yolaunda finally lost the weight she'd been struggling to lose for years...

Joan's bulimia was gone within a week...

Tom's vision improved...

Jim's shoulder pain disappeared...

Mindy's carpal tunnel syndrome went away...

Sandy's knee pain, which she had seen three other doctors for, was gone in moments...

Carol's night terrors, which had plagued her for over 30 years, were gone within a week, and did not return...

I was present at each of these events and many others like them. In many years of practice and teaching, I have seen countless seemingly miraculous healings such as these, all as a result of simply releasing trapped emotions using the Emotion Code.

My purpose in writing this book is to teach you how to find and remove trapped emotions from yourself and from others.

Whether you are a doctor or a fisherman, a housewife or a teenager, you can learn the Emotion Code. It's simple.

Anyone can learn how to be free from the very real and damaging effects of trapped emotions.

What is a Trapped Emotion?

As you live through the days and years of your life you are continually experiencing emotions of one sort or another. Life can be difficult and emotions can sometimes feel overwhelming. All of us experience negative emotional extremes at times. Most of us would rather forget some of these challenges, but unfortunately, the influence of these events can stay with us in the form of trapped emotions.

Sometimes, for reasons that we do not yet understand, emotions do not process completely. In these cases, instead of simply experiencing the emotion and then moving on, the energy of the emotion somehow becomes "trapped" within the physical body.

So instead of moving beyond your angry moment, or a temporary bout with grief or depression, this negative emotional energy can remain within your body, potentially causing significant physical and emotional stress.

Most people are amazed to find out that their "emotional baggage" is more literal than they had imagined. Trapped emotions actually consist of well-defined energies that have a shape and form. Although they are not visible, they are very real.

Neil's Resentment

In this story, a Canadian teacher shares how a difficult situation resulted in a trapped emotion that stayed with him, impacting his life in a negative way.

A number of years ago when I was teaching school, the principal and I just did not get along well at all. We fought almost from day one over one topic or another. She was extremely vicious, vindictive, and emasculating in every way, shape and form. Finally, about January of the school year, I bailed out. I saw my doctor, and went on stress leave. He said, 'Take some time off and regroup and recuperate.' So I did that for about three months, and at the end of three months I went back to the school board with a clean bill of health, but with a proviso from the doctor that I was not to be put back into the same situation with this rather nasty principal.

Anyway, the feelings surrounding her and that whole situation would never leave. They would well up often, and I would ruminate on the situation, thinking about it, and I would feel my blood pressure rising, and I would feel the anger and resentment building up within me about the way I had been treated, and the fact that she never had any disciplinary measures even though she had a history of being rather sinister, if you will, to teachers who disagreed with her approach to principalship.

Anyway, this went on for 2 years. I couldn't sleep at night because I'd be so bent out of shape from all the negative feelings I was carrying. We were visiting Southern California and went and saw Dr. Brad Nelson and went to his clinic, and he rolled a magnet up and down my back, and released this feeling of resentment, and when he did so, I felt, I actually felt, something leave me. And from that point forward, even though I still don't like the woman, I don't have the negative feelings and the rising blood pressure, the anger, the resentment, which had possessed me for several years. So, that's the story of an emotional blockage gone, with these principles and the Emotion Code that Dr. Brad teaches.

Neil B., Alberta, Canada

Your Future Held Hostage

Do you ever feel that you are struggling under the weight of something that you can't quite put your finger on? Perhaps your life is not turning out how you had hoped. Perhaps your attempts to form lasting relationships never seem to work out. You may wish that certain events in your past had never occurred but feel powerless to move beyond them. You may even have an uneasy feeling that your present is being held hostage by your past in some vague and indefinable way.

Jennifer's Self-Sabotage

Jennifer's experience is a good example of how trapped emotions can get in your way. She was my daughter's close friend, a fun-loving college student with a bright future. On her way home for the summer, she stopped by to visit our family. Her college life was going well, but she expressed concern that events from her past still troubled her, and she wondered if she was suffering from trapped emotions.

She told me she'd been involved in a tumultuous relationship with a young man the year before. Jennifer said that since the failure of that stormy relationship, she felt the sting of insecurity every time she met someone new, and had an unfounded fear of commitment that she couldn't overcome. She told me that she seemed to unintentionally sabotage every potential relationship that she began. I tested her and discovered that there was indeed, at least one trapped emotion that was contributing to her problem.

I decided to help her learn to treat herself, so she could continue to release her own trapped emotions without my assistance, since she lived some distance away. She quickly and easily learned the Emotion Code and proceeded to find several trapped emotions in her body, most notably the emotion of creative insecurity. This particular emotion arises from a lack of confidence about creating things; from painting a picture, starting a new job, or entering into a new relationship, etc. Jennifer had experienced this emotion in her prior relationship, and it had become trapped within her. She was able to release the creative insecurity as well as a few other trapped emotions from her body within a few minutes, and then continue her drive home.

A few days later she called, exclaiming that she felt an amazing difference. She said that she felt a noticeable improvement in her ability to articulate her thoughts and express herself in the company of a particular young man that she was dating. Previously she had felt intimidated and shy around him, but after releasing her trapped emotions she felt very at ease and confident. Months later, she continued to watch the relationship grow. She felt certain that she would have sabotaged it if she had not released her trapped emotions.

Getting rid of your trapped emotions can help you to overcome the obstacles of your past and can bring new life to your marriage, family, and other personal relationships.

Freeing yourself from your trapped emotions can make you feel more secure and motivated, and can liberate you to create the relationships, career, and life that you always wanted.

People frequently sense that they are somehow burdened by their past emotions, but they don't seem to know how to get over them. Some seek help through traditional psychotherapy, which does not directly address trapped emotions, but typically addresses their symptoms.

Many people fail to perform up to their ability and have difficulty making their life work as they should. Oftentimes, the underlying cause of their frustration is a trapped emotion from a past event that they may not realize is sabotaging their efforts. The next story is a perfect example of how this can happen.

Julia the Court Recorder

Julia was going to school to become a court recorder, and was excited about her future job prospects. Court recorders learn to type on a specialized phonetic machine, and have to type very rapidly and accurately to record everything said in the courtroom. Julia did fine in class, but whenever she had to take an examination where the pressure was really on, she would fail. She was very worried, as she had failed the test 3 times, and was afraid that this next examination would be her last chance to pass.

I tested her to see if there was a trapped emotion that might be influencing her behavior in the testing situation, and the answer her body gave was "Yes." In her case, the trapped emotion was discouragement. When she was 15 years old she had gone through a difficult time when her parents were divorcing. She had experienced overwhelming discouragement which had become trapped in her body. In the testing situation, with the pressure on, the trapped emotion of discouragement would sabotage her performance. We released the trapped discouragement, and she sailed through her next test feeling relaxed and confident, and received a nearly perfect score.

Julia had no idea that her parents' divorce and her old feelings about it could be affecting her negatively in the present.

In the same way that the effects of the wind are felt rather than seen, trapped emotions are invisible, yet can exert a powerful influence upon you.

It is my experience that a significant percentage of physical illness, emotional difficulty and self-sabotage are actually caused by these unseen energies.

The Emotion Code will help you reclaim your life, enjoy better health, and finally be free from the insidious and subtle forces that trapped emotions are exerting upon you.

The Damage Trapped Emotions Cause

Trapped emotions can cause you to make the wrong assumptions, overreact to innocent remarks, misinterpret behavior and short-circuit your relationships. Even worse, trapped emotions can create depression, anxiety and other unwanted feelings that you can't seem to shake. They can interfere with proper function of your body's organs and tissues, wreaking havoc with your physical health, causing pain, fatigue and illness. Yet, no matter how great your suffering may be, the invisible energy of trapped emotions will remain undiagnosed by conventional medicine, even though they may be a major causative factor in your physical and emotional difficulties.

To eliminate any kind of problem that has to do with your health or well-being, the underlying causes of the problem must be addressed. There are many powerful drugs that can relieve the symptoms of disease. But when the drug wears off, the symptoms often return, because the underlying causes of the disease have not been dealt with.

It is important for you to recognize and remove your own trapped emotions before they cause more damage. You can live a much better life by getting rid of them.

This book proclaims the truth, that trapped emotions are a significant yet hidden cause of much illness and suffering, both emotional and physical in nature.

Times Heals All Wounds? Perhaps Not...

You've probably heard it said that time heals all wounds, but this is not necessarily true. You may think you have let go of all your emotional pain from prior relationships, and maybe you've had therapy to deal with it. It may seem like it's all behind you now, but your body can literally be inhabited by the invisible energies of old emotions. These are wounds that time alone cannot and will not heal. They can cause you to act and feel differently in your current relationships and may even cause you to sabotage them.

When a trapped emotion is released, a burden is literally lifted. In fact, people often experience a feeling of lightness upon the release of a trapped emotion.

Finding and releasing those trapped negative energies can literally make changes in how you feel and behave, in the choices that you make, and in the results that you get.

The Emotion Code is about clearing away the baggage, so that you can be who you really are inside. You are not your emotional baggage, but sometimes your trapped emotions can derail you, or cause you to travel on paths you'd rather not take. Trapped emotions can keep you from living the vibrant, healthy life you are meant to live.

Trapped Emotions and Physical Pain

In addition to obvious emotional pain, millions of people are suffering from physical aches and pains. Many times there are unseen trapped emotional energies that contribute to or create physical pain.

The next example illustrates how trapped emotions can exert an astonishingly powerful influence over the physical body.

Debbie's Broken Heart

Debbie had been a patient of mine for a year or so, when one day she came into my office complaining of what she thought might be a heart attack. She had chest pain and difficulty breathing; her left arm was completely numb, as was the left side of her face. She said it had been gradually getting worse for about 24 hours. I immediately had her lie down and put my staff on alert that we may need medical assistance. After checking her vital signs and finding them to be normal, I tested her body to see if these symptoms were being caused by a trapped emotion. The answer her body gave was "Yes."

I continued to test Debbie, and quickly determined that the trapped emotion was heartache. A little more testing revealed that this emotion had become trapped in her body three years earlier. At this point she burst into tears and exclaimed, "I thought I'd dealt with all that in therapy! I can't believe that is showing up now!" I asked, "Can you share what happened?"

She replied that three years before, her husband had an affair. The news was devastating to her. It destroyed her marriage and wrecked her life for a while, but she gradually came to terms with it. She cried a lot of tears, spent a year in therapy, got remarried, and moved on- or so she thought.

Debbie expressed surprise that her past heartache was still affecting her, and in such a dramatic way. How could this event be the source of her physical pain when she'd gone to such lengths to deal with it already? She had done all the things we're told to do. She'd cried and expressed her feelings, sought the comfort of friends and the advice of therapists, opened up a dialogue with her husband and reconciled with her divorce. It had not been easy and she'd made a lot of important progress. In her mind she'd dealt with it and put it behind her.

What she didn't see is what none of us can see. There was a physical effect from her experience that was silent and invisible until she began to manifest symptoms from it. She had dealt with her troubles in every way but this. She was suffering from a trapped emotion.

I released the trapped heartache from her body, and within seconds the feeling came back into her arm and into her face. Suddenly she could breathe freely and the chest pain and heaviness were gone. She left the office shortly after, feeling completely fine.

The overwhelming heartache that she had felt during those early days of her breakup had literally become trapped in her physical body. The instantaneous relief of her physical symptoms was astounding to me. I was left to ponder on the mechanism that was at work here. How could a single trapped emotion cause such extreme physical symptoms?

Debbie's experience is a dramatic example of how trapped emotions can affect us physically, and how traditional therapy cannot and does not attempt to remove them, although traditional therapy certainly has its place. Typically trapped emotions will not cause symptoms as intense as the ones that Debbie experienced. Most are more subtle, yet exert an imbalancing influence on both mind and body.

Sharon's Mother was a Pain

A patient named Sharon came to my office one day complaining of pain in her abdomen. She told me that the pain felt like it was coming from her right ovary. I tested her to see if the cause of her pain was due to a trapped emotion, and found that it was.

Further testing revealed that the exact emotion was frustration, that it had to do with her mother, and that it had become trapped in her body three days earlier. The moment I arrived at this determination, she became quite upset and angrily hissed, "Oh, my mother! She called me three days ago, and dumped all of this stuff on me! I wish she would just get out of my life, and leave me alone!"

I released the trapped frustration from her body and the pain instantly vanished. Sharon was amazed, and could hardly believe that the pain was entirely and suddenly gone. Even more amazing to Sharon was the fact that her intense frustration with her mother was the apparent cause of the physical pain she had been suffering from for the last three days.

Trapped emotions can even create muscular imbalances that lead to joint malfunction and eventual joint degeneration and arthritis. I have seen hundreds of cases where acute physical pain instantly left the body upon the release of a trapped emotion.

Jim's Bad Knees

Removing trapped emotions can often relieve pain and suffering, even in cases that would be considered hopeless by conventional medicine. This is a letter I received from a former patient whose case certainly fits this description.

I was your patient for a few years and know that I had many physical problems with my legs, knees and back when I came to you. I was able to withstand the side effects of the various supplements you prescribed to cleanse my system and then through your abilities to release the resentments, anger and fear that I was hanging on to, we were able to achieve a physical position where my knees stopped hurting (I had been told by my doctor that replaced my hips that my knees needed replacing because they were worn out also) and I was able to walk, climb stairs, etc. pain-free for the first time in years. To this day I am basically active and pain-free. This is not to say that arthritis doesn't come into play as I continue to grow older, but the worn-out knees are still working fine and for that I am grateful. I wish you the best with your book and pray that it can open the door for others to a healthy life.

Keep the faith, Jim H.

People often put up with their pain, and end up simply "living with it", especially when they cannot find a solution or a reason for it. Pain is the body's way of telling you there is a problem; it's a warning sign.

In my experience working with people in pain, I've observed that trapped emotions are actually creating the pain at least 50% of the time.

Pinned to the Past

I was teaching a workshop once in Las Vegas when I had an interesting experience. I asked for a volunteer, and a young woman in her early twenties came up out of the audience. I asked her if she had any particular physical complaints, and she said no, that she was healthy, and had no problems.

I muscle tested her to see if she had a trapped emotion, and she did. The emotion was unsupported, which is a feeling similar to being all alone, and without help when you really need it.

Through muscle testing I asked her body when this emotion had become trapped. I asked, "Did this emotion become trapped within the last five years?" "No." "Did this emotion become trapped between ages ten and twenty?" "No." "Did this emotion become trapped between ages birth to ten?" "Yes." "Did this emotion become trapped in the first five years of your life?" "Yes." "Did this emotion become trapped in the first year of your life?" "Yes." "Did this emotion occur after one year of age?" "No." I asked her if she had any idea what this might be about, and she shook her head no.

It just so happened that this young woman had arrived at the workshop with her mother and they had been sitting together in the audience. At this point, I looked out at the audience and noticed that her mother looked very uncomfortable.

Her hand was covering her mouth and she looked either frightened or very embarrassed, I couldn't tell which. I asked her if she knew what might have happened, since her daughter was too young to remember.

In a very pained and embarrassed voice she explained, "Well, when Jessica was a baby I used cloth diapers, which I would close with safety pins. There was one particular occasion where I'm ashamed to say that I accidently pinned her to her diaper. She cried and cried, but I didn't realize that she was pinned to her diaper until I changed her again. I can't believe this is showing up now and I felt so horrible about this and I still do."

I turned to Jessica and asked, "Is that what this trapped emotion is about?" I pressed down on her arm and it was very strong, indicating that this was indeed the case. I released the trapped emotional energy by rolling three times down her back with a magnet, and she sat down again. About two weeks later I received the following e-mail:

Hi Dr. Brad,

When you were in Las Vegas, you cleared a trapped emotion for my daughter, Jessica, stemming from infancy. Jessica has suffered from hip and knee pain since about the age of 12 years...it has gotten worse as she got older. Since you worked on clearing her trapped emotion of feeling unsupported (about 1 1/2 weeks ago), she has had no pain or constriction in her hips and knees. She has never gone more than a day or two without pain, and because it was worsening, it was beginning to affect her gait. She is ecstatic, and now is experiencing a "new" sense of inner joy. She sends her heartfelt thanks.

Jessica said feel free to share her story....she is certainly telling everyone in Las Vegas about it!

Thank you! - Maureen C.

Here is another example of a trapped emotion creating physical pain. The event that caused the trapped emotion happened when Jessica was a baby, and she had no conscious memory of it. Had we not released it, I believe that Jessica may have eventually become disabled, and the true cause of her disability — her trapped emotion — would have remained undiscovered.

Of course, not all physical pain is caused by trapped emotions. But isn't it interesting to contemplate that they can cause or contribute to physical pain?

I have come to understand that trapped emotions seem to be involved, to one degree or another, in nearly every illness I have encountered. How is this possible?

Trapped Emotions and Disease

The most ancient idea in the art of healing is that disease is caused by imbalance in the body. Trapped emotions are perhaps the most common type of imbalance that human beings suffer from. I believe that trapped emotions can be implicated in nearly all diseases, either directly or indirectly.

Because trapped emotions are nearly universal, and because they always create distortion in the energy field of the body, and because they are completely invisible, they can cause an incredibly wide variety of physical problems without being unmasked.

Trapped emotions are truly epidemic, and are the insidious, invisible cause of much suffering and illness, both physical and emotional in nature.

Trapped emotions lower immune function and make the body more vulnerable to disease. They can distort body tissues, block the flow of energy, and prevent normal function of organs and glands.

On the following page is a list of conditions and diseases that my patients came to me with, where trapped emotions appeared as a contributing factor, and many times as the entire cause of the condition.

Acid Reflux	Diabetes	Learning Disabilities
ADD/ADHD	Dyslexia	Low Back Pain
Allergies	Eye Pain	Hypothyroidism
Abdominal Pain	Fibromyalgia	Lupus
Asthma	Frigidity	Migraines
Back Pain	Headaches	Multiple Sclerosis
Bell's Palsy	Heartburn (GERD)	Neck pain
Cancer	Hip Pain	Night Terrors
Carpal Tunnel	Hypoglycemia	Panic Attacks
Chest Pain	Impotency	Parkinson's disease
Chronic Fatigue	Infertility	Phobias
Chron's Disease	Insomnia	Shoulder pain
Colitis	Irritable Bowel (IBS)	Sinus problems
Constipation	Joint Pain	Tennis Elbow
Depression	Knee Pain	Vertigo

I am not saying that releasing trapped emotions is a cure-all. The Emotion Code should not be used by itself in attempting to address any major disease or medical condition, but rather, it should be looked upon as an adjunctive therapy. When trapped emotions are contributing to physical illness, removing them can only help.

The Emotion Code is easy to use and precise. Sometimes the release of a trapped emotion will bring about an instantaneous and dramatic effect, but most of the time the effects are more subtle, yet they always seem to bring a greater sense of contentment and peace, whether they are immediate or gradual.

If you are like many of the people who have come to my seminars over the years, using the Emotion Code will bring a new joy and freedom to your life.

It will give you a greater feeling of serenity because you will be freeing yourself from your old emotional baggage. The results can bring balance, a new inner calm and profound healing where nothing else has before.

THE DOCTOR OF THE FUTURE WILL GIVE NO MEDICINE,
BUT WILL INTEREST HIS PATIENTS IN THE CARE
OF THE HUMAN FRAME, IN DIET, AND IN
THE CAUSE AND PREVENTION OF DISEASE.

- THOMAS A. EDISON

2

THE SECRET WORLD OF TRAPPED EMOTIONS

By now, you are probably wondering whether you have any trapped emotions yourself, and what they might be. Here is a list of circumstances that often result in trapped emotions:

- Loss of a loved one
- Divorce or relationship problems
- Financial hardship
- Home or work stress
- Miscarriage or Abortion
- Physical trauma
- Physical or Emotional Combat
- Physical, mental, verbal or sexual abuse
- Negative self-talk
- Negative beliefs about yourself or others

- Long-term stress
- Rejection
- Physical illness
- Feelings of inferiority
- Internalization of feelings
- Neglect or abandonment

This list is by no means all-inclusive. The only way to know whether you have trapped emotions is to ask the subconscious mind. This can be done quite easily, but first a little explanation is in order.

Conscious versus Subconscious

First, let's discuss the difference between the conscious and the subconscious mind.

Here is a simple way to look at it. It has been said many times that we humans use only about 10% of our brain. What is really meant by this is that the conscious mind needs about 10% of our brain's resources. In other words, thinking, moving about, making choices, planning, seeing, hearing, tasting, touching, and smelling are all conscious activities, and take up 10% of the processing power of our brain.

If this is true, what is the other 90% of the brain doing? If the conscious mind takes up 10% of your brain, we can refer to the other 90% as the subconscious mind. This silent and unconscious majority of the brain is constantly busy storing information and keeping your body systems running efficiently. It is also important to understand that the subconscious mind exerts an unseen, yet profound influence over the things we do, and how we behave and feel.

Most people give little thought to their subconscious minds. But imagine for a moment having to take over the functions that your subconscious mind performs. Imagine the difficulty of instructing your digestive system how to digest your lunch, or telling your cells how to create enzymes and proteins. Imagine if you had to worry about keeping your heart beating or keeping air moving in and out of your lungs every moment of every day. And you think you have a full schedule now!

Like a computer, your subconscious mind is capable of storing vast amounts of information.

Brain surgery is often done while the patient is conscious. The brain has no pain-sensing nerves, and surgeons take advantage of this fact to get feedback from their patients while their brains are being delicately probed during surgery.

 Dr. Wilder Penfield discovered that under certain circumstances people who are undergoing brain surgery will have memories return to them when a certain area of the brain is stimulated. For example, the surgeon might touch an area of the brain with his electrode and the alert patient suddenly will remember a scene, a smell, or a sound from a particular moment in their life.[1]

Often these flashes of memory are about events or scenes that would be unremembered under normal circumstances. If the same area of the brain is touched again with an electrode in the same precise spot, the same memory will be reexperienced.

If you are like me, sometimes it seems difficult to remember what happened yesterday. I believe, however, that your subconscious mind is an amazing recording device.

I believe that everything you've ever done in your entire life has been logged in your subconscious mind.

Every face you've ever seen in a crowd, every smell, every voice, every song, every taste, every touch and every sensation you have ever experienced has been recorded by your subconscious.

Every virus, bacteria or fungus that has ever invaded your body, all your injuries, all your thoughts and feelings, and the entire history of every cell in your body has all been archived. Your subconscious is also aware of any trapped emotions that your body may be harboring, and it also knows exactly what effect these trapped emotions are having on your physical,

---

1 Jefferson Lewis, Something Hidden: A Biography of Wilder Penfield (Goodread Biographies), (Halifax, Nova Scotia: Formac Publishing Company Ltd., 1951), 198.

emotional and mental well-being. All of this and more is tucked away in the subconscious mind.

The Computer-Mind

Your subconscious is also aware of exactly what your body needs in order to get well. But how can you get to this information?

I began asking myself that same question when I was in chiropractic school. I learned that the brain is essentially a computer, the most powerful computer in the known universe. This made me wonder if healers would ever be able to tap into the immense power of the brain, to find critical information about what was wrong with their patients.

During my years of practice, I learned that it is actually possible to retrieve information from the subconscious, using a form of kinesiology, or muscle testing. First developed by Dr. George Goodheart in the 1960s as a way to correct structural imbalance in the skeleton, muscle testing is now widely accepted. While many physicians world-wide use muscle testing procedures to correct spinal misalignments and other imbalances, the fact that muscle testing can be used to get information directly from the subconscious mind is less recognized.[2]

---

2 Robert Frost, *Applied Kinesiology: A Training Manual and Reference Book of Basic Principles and Practice*, (Berkeley, CA: North Atlantic Books, 2002), 4.

Talking to the Body

The ability to open a line of communication with a patient's subconscious mind through muscle testing became a powerful tool for me. It enabled me to know what a patient needed in order to get well, as quickly as possible. I came to trust the body's wisdom implicitly and to have great faith in the body's innate ability to communicate that wisdom to me, through muscle testing. Many years of teaching seminars to both lay-people and doctors taught me that anyone can do it. Anyone can learn to get answers from the body, and anyone can take the necessary steps to help the body heal. You don't have to be a doctor; you just have to be willing to learn.

I have been driven for many years to share this marvelous knowledge with the world. It took much prayer and effort to refine and simplify the Emotion Code, and now it is simple enough that anyone can learn it. You will soon have all the knowledge you need to begin using this method on yourself to remove trapped emotional energies from your body.

Negative versus Positive Stimuli

Before I can teach you how to get information from your subconscious mind, you must understand one basic principle. This is that all organisms, no matter how primitive, will respond to positive or negative stimuli. For example, plants grow towards sunlight and away from darkness. An amoeba in an aquarium will move towards light and away from darkness. If a drop of poison is placed into that same aquarium, the amoeba will move away from that poison and head toward cleaner water.

On a subconscious level, the human body is no different.

Your body will normally be drawn toward positive things or thoughts and repelled by negative things or ideas.

In fact, this has been going on all your life, without your even being aware of it. If you will allow yourself to quiet your conscious mind and tune in to your body, you will learn that your subconscious is quite able to communicate with you.

Are you ready to let your subconscious mind speak to you?

The Sway Test

The simplest method I know of to get answers from your subconscious mind is called the Sway Test. You will learn other methods of muscle testing later on in this book, but the Sway Test is extremely simple to learn and does not require the assistance of anyone else, and so can be used when you are alone.

To try the Sway Test, assume a standing position and make sure you are comfortable. The room should be quiet and free of distractions, including music and television. It will be easiest for you to learn if you are alone or with someone who is learning along with you.

Here's what to do:

Stand with your feet shoulder width apart so that you are comfortably balanced.

Stand still, with your hands by your sides.

Let go of all your worries and relax your body completely. Close your eyes if you are comfortable doing so.

Within a few seconds you will notice that it is actually impossible to stand perfectly still. Your body will continually shift its position very slightly in different directions as your muscles work to maintain your standing posture. You will notice that these movements are very slight, and are not under your conscious control.

When you make a positive, true or congruent statement, your body should begin to sway noticeably forward, usually within less than ten seconds. When you make an incongruent or untrue statement your body should sway backwards within the same time frame.

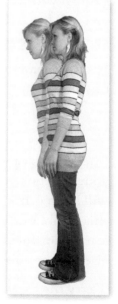

Swaying Forward

34

I believe this phenomenon occurs because of how you are used to perceiving the world around you. In spite of the fact that your environment surrounds you completely at all times, on all sides, you are used to only dealing with what is directly in front of you at any given time. When you drive a car, when you walk, when you eat, when you work at your desk, you are constantly dealing with the world in front of you, not the world behind you or to the sides of you. When you make any kind of a statement, your body perceives that thought as if it were like anything else it has to deal with, like a file on your desk or food on your plate. Essentially, you can think of the statement you make as being right in front of you, ready to be dealt with and processed.

When you are ready, simply state the words "unconditional love." Keep this phrase in your mind, and try to feel the feelings that are connected with this phrase. In a few moments, you should notice your body sway forward. Like a plant growing toward the light, your body will gently sway toward the positive energy of that thought. The movement of your body toward this thought may be more sudden than gradual in some cases, and may surprise you!

Now clear your mind, and say the word "hatred." Try to feel the feelings that are connected with this thought. Just as any organism will automatically move away from a poisonous or harmful substance, your body should move away from the thought of "hatred." You should notice that your body, within ten seconds or so, will begin to sway backward. It is very important that you don't try to force your body to sway either forward or backward. Simply allow your body to sway on its own. You are giving your subconscious mind its first opportunity to speak to you in this very direct way, and it must be done gently for the best result. Don't force it. It will become easier with practice.

Now try making a statement that you know to be true. State your name out loud, saying, "My name is _____." If your name is Alex for example, you would say, "My name is Alex." Your subconscious mind knows what is congruent or true. When you make a true statement, you'll feel your body begin to gently sway forward, because your body is drawn towards positivity, congruency and truth.

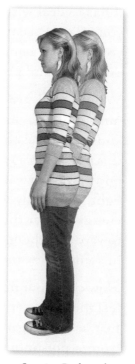

Now you can try an untrue or incongruent statement. If your name is Alex for example, you might say, "My name is Chris", or "My name is Kim." As long as you choose a name that is not your own, your subconscious mind will know that this statement is incongruent or untrue. Once you have made this statement, if you keep your mind

Swaying Backward

clear of other thoughts, you should feel your body begin to sway backwards within a few seconds. This is because your body is not only repelled by negative thoughts such as "hatred", but incongruence and falsity are also repulsive to the mind and body.

Keep Your Mind Clear

Make sure you keep your mind clear of other thoughts after making your statement. If your thoughts are wandering, it will be difficult for your subconscious mind to determine exactly what it is you are after. What if, for example, you make a positive or true statement, but then immediately begin thinking about the argument you had with your spouse last night? You will probably sway backwards, because the memory of that event is negative, and your body will naturally want to move away from it.

It is important to have patience with yourself. When you are first learning this method, it may take a little longer than expected for your body to sway. Don't get discouraged if this happens.

Your body's response time will shorten significantly the more you practice. The most challenging aspect of this form of testing for many people is that it requires them to give up control for a few moments, and allow their body to do what it wants to do. For some, giving up control is not easy. Nevertheless, this is a simple skill to learn, and it shouldn't take you very long to become proficient.

The main thing is to stay focused on whatever statement or thought you are putting out. Just keep your mind calm and allow your subconscious to communicate with you through the mechanism of your physical body.

If for any reason, you are not physically able to perform this test, don't worry. There are several other options that I will outline for you in chapter five.

Do You Have a Trapped Emotion?

As soon as you think you have the hang of it, you are ready to put the Sway Test to good use. Make this statement, "I have a trapped emotion." Your body will most likely sway forward, giving you an affirmative answer that you have at least one trapped emotion. If your body sways backward, don't assume that you are free of trapped emotions just yet. This may mean that your trapped emotions are buried a bit deeper and might take a little more effort to uncover, but it's not a problem. I will discuss how to find and release this type of trapped emotion later on.

What Trapped Emotions Are Made Of

Everything in the universe is made of energy, whether that energy manifests in physical form or remains invisible. It is the particular arrangement of these energies, and their specific rates of vibration, that determine how they will appear to us. At the most basic level, everything that exists is made of the same stuff — energy. Not only are you made of energy, but other forms of energy are passing through your body at this very moment. Energy that we cannot see is all around us in the form of radio waves, x-rays, infrared, thought waves and emotions.

We are like fish swimming in a sea of energy. Energy is the material from which all things are made; it is in all things and through all things, and fills the interspaces of the universe.

We can feel energy when it is in the form of emotions, and if negative emotional energies become trapped within us, they may adversely affect us. Trapped emotions are made of energy, just as energy makes up our bodies and everything else in the universe.

Where Our Emotions Come From

Thousands of years ago, ancient physicians were astute observers of the human body. They found that people whose lives were dominated by a certain emotion would have corresponding physical ailments. For example, people whose lives were ruled by anger seemed to suffer from liver and gall bladder trouble. People who spent their lives feeling grief would often suffer from lung or colon trouble. Fearful people seemed to have kidney and bladder problems.

Eventually, a correlation was made between the emotions we experience and the various organs of the body. It was believed that the organs themselves actually produced the emotions that people felt.

In other words, if you are feeling the emotion of fear, your kidneys or bladder are creating that particular energy or vibration. If you are feeling grief, it is being produced by your lungs or your colon, and so on.

Of course, we now know that certain areas of the brain are activated when we feel certain emotions. We also know that there is a biochemical component to the emotions that we feel. Dr. Candace Pert, in her book <u>Molecules of Emotion</u> clearly explains this biochemical side of our nature, which is perfectly valid.[3]

There is an energetic side to our nature as well, and there is an energetic component to our emotions that is only now beginning to be explored and correlated by modern science.

After much experience gained from clinical practice, I am convinced that the organs in the body really do produce the emotions we experience. The ancient physicians were right. If you're feeling an emotion of anger, it's not coming entirely from your brain; it's actually emanating from your liver or gall bladder. If you are feeling the emotion of betrayal, the emotion is emanating from your heart or your small intestine.

Remember that we used to think the body and the <u>mind were se</u>parate and distinct, but their dividing

3 Candace B. Pert, *Molecules of Emotion: Why You Feel the Way You Feel*, (New York: Touchstone Press, 1997)

line has now blurred to the point where we don't know where the influence of one begins and the other ends.

Your *entire body* is intelligent, not just your brain. Your organs are separate intelligences within your body that perform certain functions and produce specific emotions or feelings.

People are usually surprised to learn that the various organs in our bodies produce the emotions that we feel. Yet there are correlations to this principle in life that are quite distinct, although they escape the attention of most physicians.

Did Trapped Emotions Kill Dana Reeve?

We all remember the tragic injury that rendered actor Christopher Reeve a quadriplegic. We were touched by the unfailing devotion of his wife, Dana, and were shocked and saddened when she died. It was only ten months after her husband's death that she announced to the world that she had lung cancer, and seven months later she died at age 44.

Dana Reeve was a non-smoker who died of lung cancer, and although conventional wisdom holds that her death was due to second-hand smoke, I believe otherwise. The lungs produce the emotion we call grief, and an over-abundance of grief will certainly lead to the creation of trapped emotions, often affecting the parent organ. Dana certainly had reasons to grieve, and

I believe that trapped emotions, grief among others, were at least partly responsible for her death, and perhaps entirely responsible.

The Angry Drunk

Another example can be found in the way that alcohol affects people. We all know that people who become alcoholics often die of liver disease. But we also know that many people who drink can become quite angry and violent when under the influence. Alcohol is broken down and processed by the liver, and too much alcohol over-stimulates the liver. When you over-stimulate or overload an organ, it will produce more of the emotion that it is designed to produce. The liver produces feelings of anger. This is the mechanism that is often at work when drinking results in violence.

If you have an organ that is diseased, overstimulated, or imbalanced in some way, the emotions related to that organ will often be heightened.

Trapped emotions are always found to have emanated from a particular organ, no matter where that trapped emotion lodges in the body. For example, a trapped emotion of anger may have originally emanated from your liver, but it may become lodged literally anywhere in your body.

Correlations between the organs and our emotions are both fascinating and important to understanding how our bodies really work. It all goes back to the ancient art of energy healing.

Energy Medicine

Energy healing is one of the oldest practices known in the world today. Since 4000 B.C., healers have understood that our health greatly depends on the quality of energy that flows through and makes up our bodies. In Chinese medicine, that energy is called "Qi" or "Chi." In Ancient Indian or Ayurvedic medicine, this energy is called "Prana." Imbalances of this part of our existence may deeply affect our physical and mental health.

We can compare this energy to electricity. We can't see electricity, but we can feel it. Electricity is colorless and odorless. It's invisible, yet it certainly is real. If you've ever stuck your finger in a light socket or been shocked getting the toast out of a toaster, then you'll know what I mean. You may not be able to see it, but it's definitely there!

As human beings, we are used to perceiving things in a way that conforms to our belief systems. We form our beliefs about the physical world at an early age. We learn that if we fall off the monkey bars at school, we will meet the ground with a painful thud, yet we could never imagine that both the ground and the monkey bars, as solid as they seem to us, are actually made of vibrating energies. We may like to think that the world around us is exactly as we are used to seeing it, but Einstein, Tesla and others have shown us that the universe is really much more complex and wonderful than we ever could possibly have imagined.

The Quantum World

You must remember that old saying, "I know it like the back of my hand…" But how well do you really know the back of your hand?

Take a look at it. Your eyes see the surface of your skin with its wrinkles, fingernails and little hairs. You know exactly how the back of your hand looks from that perspective. But if you magnify your hand under a microscope, you won't see the same skin and creases you've become so familiar with. Instead, you might think you are looking at the surface of a strange planet, covered with hills and valleys.

Turn up the power on your microscope, magnifying your skin 20,000 times, and you'll see a field of swarming cells. Magnify it a lot more and you'll see molecules. Magnify those molecules and you'll see the atoms that make up those molecules. Magnify those atoms and you'll see the subatomic energy clouds that make up those atoms- the electrons, the protons, the neutrons and other subatomic particles. It's still the back of your hand, but it looks nothing like the hand you know.

If you glance at it now, your hand looks solid. Slap it down on the table and it makes a nice, substantial thud. Your hand may seem solid, but there's actually a lot of empty space there. At the subatomic level, there are vast distances between each spinning electron. Atoms are 99.99999999% empty space. Your hand is

99.99999999% empty space! If you could remove all the empty space from the atoms in your hand, it would become so small you would need a microscope to see it! It would virtually disappear, although it would still weigh the same and contain the same number of atoms.

It might take a moment to comprehend this idea. Your hand seems solid, but it is made of dynamic energy, in constant vibration. In fact, physicists now understand that the so-called "subatomic particles" which make up the atom are not really particles at all. They measure the contents of the atom in "energy units" instead, because it's so much more accurate.[4]

Thoughts are Energy

Like everything else in the universe, the thoughts that you create are made of energy.

Thought-energy has no boundary. Your thoughts are not confined to a certain volume and location like your physical body.

While we like to think that all of our unspoken thoughts are private and that they are confined to our own heads, it's not true.

Each of us is like a radio station, constantly broadcasting the energy of our thoughts, which emanate from us

---

4 Isaac Asimov, *Atom: Journey Across the Subatomic Cosmos* (New York: Penguin Books USA Inc., 1992), 56.

and fill the immensity of space, touching all those around us for good or ill.

This doesn't mean that we can read other people's minds, but the energy of other people's thoughts *are* detected to some degree on a subconscious level. Try staring intently at the back of someone's head in a crowd, and inevitably they will turn and look right at you before long. Lots of us have had this experience, and if you haven't, try it. It works every time!

We are all Connected

The reality is, the entire human family is connected energetically. When people are suffering and dying on the other side of the earth, we feel their distant cries and anguish on a subconscious level and we are darkened by it. When something tragic happens in the world, the whole world feels it subconsciously, and is affected by it. On the other hand, when wonderful things happen in the world, we all are brightened together.

The connectedness that we all have will often manifest as subtle thoughts that float up from the subconscious level to our conscious minds.

This energy connection seems strongest between a mother and her children. Mothers often seem to be able to sense when one of their children is in trouble. We call this mother's intuition, and my own mother was an expert at it. Our connection to our own mothers is perhaps strongest because of the spiritual umbilical that binds us to them.

The most powerful example of this energetic connection occurred to one of my patients a number of years ago. She was sitting at home one night, watching television with her husband. Suddenly, she began experiencing severe, hammering pains throughout her body which inexplicably moved from one area to another. The violence of this sudden attack was terrifying, and when it was over she was greatly relieved, but exhausted and frightened. She had never experienced anything like this before, and had no idea what had suddenly gone wrong in her body. Her attempts to explain this bizarre and excruciating attack baffled everyone, including her doctors.

Three days later, she got a phone call from her son, who was working in the Philippines. He called her from his hospital bed and told her that he had been severely beaten by the local police a few days before. When they compared the time of his beating to the time of her experience, they were one and the same. Somehow, she was connected enough to her son to literally "feel his pain." Talk about mother's intuition!

Thoughts are Powerful

Your thoughts are immensely powerful. Whenever you say what you're thinking or write something down, you're using the energy of your thoughts to affect the world around you. It is through thought, belief and intention that all things happen.

Reputable laboratory experiments have repeatedly shown that thoughts can directly influence the rate of growth in plants, fungi, and bacteria. William Tiller, a physicist at Stanford University, has shown that thoughts can affect electronic instruments.[5]

Studies have proven that when the energy of thought is directed intentionally, it can impact someone else, regardless of whether they are nearby or all the way around the world.

Depending on whether the person focusing the thought uses calming or activating imagery, for instance, they can create a greater sense of relaxation or anxiety in the targeted person. The effect is so distinctive that it can be measured in a laboratory by galvanic skin response, a highly sensitive method of measuring electrical changes in the skin.[6]

Imagine how your own thoughts affect you. Everyone has some kind of internal conversation at times. What do you say to yourself? Many people criticize themselves far more often than they praise themselves. Negative self-talk may be hurting you more than you realize.

5 William A. Tiller, Walter E. Dibble, Jr. and Michael J. Kohane, *Conscious Acts of Creation: The Emergence of a New Physics* (Walnut Creek, CA: Pavior Publishing, 2001),1.
6 William A. Tiller, *Science and Human Transformation: Subtle Energies, Intention-ality and Consciousness* (Walnut Creek, CA: Pavior Publishing, 1997), 14.

What about other people around you? Do you ever wonder if others can sense how you feel about them? Other people's subconscious minds are continually detecting the vibrations of your thoughts. Have you ever had a moment with a friend, where he or she blurted out just what you were thinking? Have you ever instinctively known who was about to call you, before the phone even rang? These are not coincidences, they are evidences of the power of thought energy.

Finding trapped emotions using the Emotion Code is along the same lines as detecting the vibration of another person's thoughts or feelings. The difference is that you can ask the body, and actually get definitive answers, instead of guessing. Then you can release the trapped emotions for good, and know with certainty that they are permanently gone.

Serendipity vs Precision

Any alternative health care practitioner can tell you that almost everyone carries around old emotional energies from their past. Our physical bodies hold onto trapped emotions, and doctors and body workers are aware of this because often a simple touch can bring out a flood of emotions and memories in a patient. At one time or another, nearly every practitioner I know — from chiropractors to energy workers to massage therapists — has had the experience of provoking an unexpected emotional release in a patient, as the body let go of the energy it had been holding on to. Releasing those trapped emotions can result in profound and immediate healing. While any emotional release that occurs in this serendipitous way is welcome, this is usually not the intention of the therapist, and any emotional release that occurs is only accidental.

The Emotion Code approach, however, is much more deliberate. I sometimes think of it as "emotional surgery" because we are searching out the trapped emotions with a clear intention of removing them. Nothing is left to chance. Trapped emotions are potentially so destructive that you need to find them and get them out of your body, and then confirm that they have been released. The Emotion Code helps you do exactly that in a precise and simple way.

Trapped Emotions and Children

I have twin boys who are, at the time of this writing, eighteen years old. One of my early experiences with trapped emotions happened with my son, Rhett when he was a toddler. Rhett and Drew are fraternal twins, and are about as different as two boys can be. Drew was always very affectionate with both my wife and me. Rhett was very affectionate with my wife Jean, but developed some sort of hang-up about me around age three. When I would try to hug him or be close to him or snuggle with him he would push me away and say "Bad doctor! Away!" At first we thought he was just passing through some kind of stage. We assumed that he would grow out of it, but his negative feelings toward me persisted for over a year. It was a source of heartache and frustration to me. I didn't understand why my little boy felt this way about me.

One evening, Jean and I were sitting and talking together. Rhett was sitting on Jean's lap. I opened my arms to him to give him a hug. He gave me the same reaction as before, pushing me away and saying "Bad doctor! Away!" This time I really felt the hurt. I could feel the heartache welling up within my chest, and I felt like I was going to cry. My wife said, "You know, maybe he has a trapped emotion."

Up until this point we had only treated adults for trapped emotions. We decided to check him and see. Using the Emotion Code we found that he did have a trapped emotion. The emotion was grief. But it wasn't his grief about me, it was actually my grief about him. In other words, at some point he perceived that I had grief about him. He felt that grief strongly enough that it created a trapped emotion in his body. Testing showed that this emotion became trapped when my oldest daughter and I had an argument that Rhett was witness to. Even though I was not grieved about him, he perceived the grief I was experiencing about her, and applied it to himself.

We released the trapped grief, and to my amazement he walked right over to me and put his arms around me. As I cried and held my little boy, I was astonished and excited at the same time. If my son could be changed so instantaneously by simply removing a trapped emotion, then how many other children could be helped?

The Pilot's Daughter

The next day in my clinic I was talking with a patient about what had happened with Rhett. She said, "You know, I think my little girl might have a trapped emotion. My husband is an airline pilot. Every week he's gone for several days in a row, and when he comes back, our six-year-old daughter will run and hide from him. She just won't have anything to do with him when he comes home from his trips, and it breaks his heart."

She brought her daughter into the office the following day. I found that she did have a trapped emotion about her father. In this case, the trapped emotion was sorrow. It was her own sorrow about her father leaving and being gone for long periods of time. At some point, this sorrow was so strong that it imbalanced her body, and the emotion became trapped. This emotional energy was exerting a very strong subconscious affect and was influencing her behavior towards him. We released the emotion, and they went home.

The following week the mother returned to the office and said, "Doctor Nelson, your emotional treatment really works. My husband was gone when I came in and had my daughter treated. A few days ago my husband came home from overseas, and when he opened the door our little girl ran and jumped into his arms. She has never done that, ever! He is thrilled! Thank you so much."

Drew and His Traumatic Delivery

By the time our twin boys were four years old, Rhett was very articulate and talkative. Drew was just the opposite, so much so that my wife and I began to grow concerned. At four years old, Drew still wasn't speaking in sentences. He rarely said a word and when he started to speak he'd often put his hand over his mouth, as though he were afraid to say anything.

He seemed fearful in general. When we went to the neighborhood pool, Rhett jumped right in, but Drew stood at the edge, looking anxious. He was very cautious about trying new things. He was also claustrophobic. If he went outside to play and the door closed behind him, he would panic and scream.

Psychological testing showed that Drew had a high IQ, but was not developing at the same pace as the norm for other kids his age. Hearing tests showed that his hearing was normal. There seemed to be no explanation for what was going on with Drew.

After our experience with Rhett, we decided to see if Drew might have trapped emotions, not realizing that they were the actual cause of his troubles.

As we tested him, we quickly found a number of trapped emotions that were the result of traumatic things that had happened on the day that he was born and shortly thereafter.

Jean's labor and delivery had been very long, lasting twenty-two hours total. Rhett was born first. He looked beautiful and content and immediately went to sleep. Drew was born 14 minutes later and emerged blue and limp, looking really rough. A team of doctors circled around him immediately. They weren't sure he would make it. His situation was critical.

He pulled through, but the next 10 days or so continued to be very traumatic. We had taken both of the boys home when they were a couple of days old but Drew had to be readmitted to the hospital for testing to see what was wrong. He was unable to keep any breast milk down and was rapidly loosing weight. We were told that he had picked up a life-threatening infection during his first few days. The doctors had to do a spinal tap on his tiny body, and administer antibiotics intravenously to save his life.

Against our wishes, Jean and I were ordered out of the room as this procedure was begun. We were unable to comfort him in any way, and could only listen helplessly as Drew screamed in terror while they repeatedly tried to insert the needles into his tiny veins and into his spine.

We didn't dwell on Drew's traumatic experiences ourselves, and we never discussed these events with him as a child. It was very upsetting for us to even think about it. Four years later, as far as we knew, he had no memory of these events, but he did have a lot of fear, about a lot of things.

One by one, we found and released the trapped emotions that related to these traumatic events. We were amazed by what Drew had perceived as an infant, and how deeply it had scarred him emotionally. He probably expected that coming into the world would be wonderful. Instead he came into an incredibly painful situation that he could scarcely cope with. It was like being born into hell. As you might imagine, he had trapped emotions of fear, terror and abandonment. Undoubtedly, these were the exact feelings he'd had during the emergency room procedures that we all found so difficult to endure.

Drew had also developed a trapped emotion of panic while he was in the womb waiting in line behind his reluctant brother, who was in no hurry to emerge from his dark and comfortable home. This trapped emotion of panic proved to be the reason behind his claustrophobia.

In addition, he had a trapped emotion of anger that he had *inherited* from his grandfather. It was actually this inherited anger that was making him reluctant to talk. He was afraid that he would hurt someone with his words, which explained why he would always cover his mouth when he would speak. We released all of these trapped emotions and retired for the night.

The next morning at breakfast, we couldn't believe the difference! Drew was like a little chatterbox. Suddenly and for the first time in his life, he was speaking in complete sentences. Without the trapped emotions keeping him attached to the traumas of the past, he was able to let go of his fears. His claustrophobia vanished, along with his fearful attitude. He was free to become bright, happy, and inquisitive.

Trapped Emotions are Common

It isn't really possible to tell by looking at someone if they have trapped emotions, but nearly everyone does. During my years in practice, it was rare that I treated a patient who had no discernible trapped emotions. I remember one patient in particular who fell into this category. This man spent a lot of time in meditation, and struck me as being a calm, kind and unflappable sort of person who was very much in control of his emotions. Did I say "in control of his emotions?" We will talk more about that very subject in chapter ten, in terms of avoiding trapped emotions in the future.

The vast majority of us do have trapped emotions, simply because of what we have been through and who we are at this point in our journey.

Often, when someone has been through a traumatic or intensely emotional event — such as a car accident, an argument or a divorce — they will have trapped emotional energy about it. However, not every emotional event will create a trapped emotion. The body is designed to deal with emotional energy in the normal course of events. So when an emotion becomes trapped, it's partly because of extenuating circumstances — such as when we have lowered resistance or when we are overly tired or otherwise off-balance. When our bodies are not at their best we are more vulnerable to developing trapped emotions.

The Resonance of Trapped Emotions

Each trapped emotion resides in a specific location in the body, vibrating at its own particular frequency. Before long, that vibration will cause surrounding tissues to vibrate at that same frequency. We call this phenomenon *resonance*.

In my seminars, I use tuning forks to demonstrate how powerfully our universe responds to resonance. One of my tuning forks vibrates at 512 Hz. The sound it makes is very high-pitched. The tines of the other tuning fork are a different size. That fork vibrates at 128 HZ and makes a much lower sound.

If you were to place any number of different-sized tuning forks in a room, and strike one of them, all the other tuning forks of that particular frequency would start humming faintly. If you stop the sound coming from the tuning fork you struck, all the others will keep vibrating. It's not because of some natural affinity between tuning forks. This is the way our universe works.

If you strike a tuning fork and place it against a pane of glass, the glass will begin to vibrate at the same frequency. That's because the tuning fork forces the energies that make up the glass into motion – in sync with its own vibration. When you have a trapped emotion it's a bit like having a tuning fork in your body that is continually vibrating at the

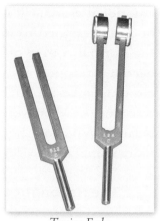

Tuning Forks

specific frequency of a negative emotion. Unfortunately this may bring more of this particular emotion into your life.

Have you ever seen someone who's agitated infect a roomful of people with that same emotion? Maybe you're calmly waiting in a doctor's office with several other people who are quietly reading magazines, when an upset patient comes in. He paces around the room, picking up magazines, then putting them back down. He speaks to the receptionist in an irritated tone. His body language gives his mood away. But it's the invisible effect that's most powerful.

That patient is sending a strong, agitated vibration out into the room. Some of the cells in your body and those of the receptionist and the other patients will literally start vibrating at that frequency. Before long, everyone's feeling a little agitated. It changes the mood of the room. People start feeling differently and reacting differently. The agitated patient has not only attracted more agitation into his own life. He's actually generated it in the people around him as well.

Negative Vibrations

If you have a trapped emotion, you will attract more of that emotion into your life. You will also tend to feel that emotion more readily and more often than you otherwise would.

You can think of a trapped emotion as being like a ball of energy, because that is exactly what it is. They have a size and a shape, even though they are invisible and are made only of energy. They usually seem to vary in size from that of an orange to that of a melon.

Trapped emotional energy will always lodge somewhere in the physical body, and the body tissues that lie within that sphere will tend to fall into resonance with the vibrational energy of the trapped emotion. In other words, those tissues will actually be experiencing that emotional vibration on a continual basis.

Suppose you have a trapped emotion of anger. You've carried it around for years, not even knowing it was there. As a result, whenever you come into a situation where you *could* become angry, it's much more likely that you *will* become angry, because in a fascinating and literal way, part of you is *already* angry.

If part of your body is *already* vibrating at the frequency of anger due to a trapped emotion, it is much easier for your entire being to fall into resonance with anger when something happens that *could* elicit an angry response from you.

Sometimes people don't understand why they get ticked off so easily, or why they can't shake certain emotions. It's often because the very emotion they are struggling with is trapped within them, from a past experience they may scarcely remember.

This is why, when trapped emotions are released, the effect is incomparable to any other form of therapy. Often, the emotion and behavior that has been so difficult to shake, is simply gone.

It can seem almost too simple to believe, but once you experience it yourself, you will understand. Until you release your own trapped emotions, you will continue to labor under their weight.

Lori and the Cheerleader

I have seen this phenomenon on countless occasions, but one particular patient's experience will help to illustrate this. Lori had a trapped emotion of resentment. When I traced the original occurrence of this emotion back in time, I found that it had become trapped in high school, and that it was actually her resentment for another female. At this point, Lori said, "Well, of course. I know exactly what this is about." She explained that there was a particular girl on the cheerleading squad that she just could not stand. For whatever reasons, she felt a lot of resentment for this girl during their high school years. The resentment never really went away, since it had become trapped in Lori's body.

Lori said, "You know, I still have so much resentment for her. It's kind of weird, I guess. I'm forty-three years old now. High school was a long time ago. You'd think I would have forgotten all about her, but it's like I can't let go of it. I haven't even seen her since high school, but whenever I think of her, I can just feel this resentment welling up inside of me, and I feel all that resentment for her all over again."

I explained to Lori how a trapped emotion can make it much harder for us to let go of things we would rather forget. Using a magnet, we released the trapped emotion in a few seconds, and she left the office. I saw Lori again a few days later, and she exclaimed, "Dr. Nelson, it worked! Last night I was talking with an old girlfriend, and that girl's name came up. For the first time since high school, I felt nothing! Normally, I would have felt that resentment for her, but I felt nothing! That is so great. Thanks!"

Kirk's Life-long Anger Problem

Kirk was an angry man. He came to me when he was in his late seventies for treatment of his back pain. It quickly became obvious that there was something else bothering him. He snapped at my office staff, and tended to be curt with me as well. He was dismissive with his wife, who was nothing but supportive and kind to him. At first I attributed his behavior to the fact that he was in pain. As his back began to improve, however, his behavior did not. I decided to check him for trapped emotions, and found anger, bitterness, anxiety, resentment, frustration and fear, many of which dated back to childhood.

The end result of releasing these emotions was that Kirk became a changed man. He is now a sweet and doting husband, more concerned about his wife than his own aches and pains.

He used to complain constantly about everything, and now he turns his interest to others, usually has a smile on his face and complains very little. The transformation has been remarkable to everyone that knows him. If only his trapped emotions could have been released early in his life, he might have had a different kind of life.

Kirk was always free to choose his emotional state, but his trapped emotions made it easier for him to fall into resonance with them than to go against the current. Parts of his body were angry, bitter, anxious, resentful, frustrated and fearful. That's what he was up against every waking moment of his life, until we released those energies.

The Effect of an Imbalance

It all comes back to the quantum nature of the body itself. When we get up every morning, we expect to see our bodies looking the same they did yesterday and the day before. They seem solid and predictable enough. We never glance in the mirror while we're trying to get dressed only to see swirling clouds of energy where our arms and legs used to be. But that's exactly what we are.

No matter how it may seem to you, your body is actually a collection of energies, flying in close formation.

When you introduce the negative vibration of a trapped emotion into that formation, you alter the normal vibrational rate of the whole.

You won't necessarily feel it and you definitely can't tell the difference by looking, but there are other ways to tell.

Remember the tuning fork effect. When your body is hosting a trapped emotion, it will attract other emotions that vibrate at the same frequency. If the emotion is fear, for instance, you will become more easily frightened. The longer that energy resides inside your body, the more you'll get used to feeling it. Over time, you'll start thinking you're just a fearful person, because you seem to be afraid so much of the time. In reality, because part of your body actually exists within this particular trapped emotional energy or literal "ball of fear", you are set up for failure. Part of your body is already feeling that emotion on a continual basis so you will much more readily fall into a state of fear when a fearful situation presents itself. In other words, since part of your body is already resonating at the frequency of fear, it's a small step for your entire body to fall into resonance.

Where Trapped Emotions Lodge

People often ask me why an emotion gets trapped in one area of the body and not another. I often find that trapped emotions lodge in an area that's vulnerable because of a genetic susceptibility, an injury or nutritional deficiency that weakens or imbalances the energy of the body in that area.

Sometimes there's a metaphor at work as well. This makes sense when you realize that our subconscious minds govern our bodies and our dreams.

Symbols and metaphors are the language of the subconscious mind, so it's very natural for trapped emotions to lodge in an area that has symbolic significance.

For example, let's say you're experiencing grief for a friend who has had a miscarriage. Instead of experiencing the emotion and leaving it behind, the emotion becomes trapped. It wouldn't be surprising for that trapped emotion to lodge in your womb or breast – the nourishing organs of creation. Or suppose you're experiencing one of those difficult periods in life where a series of things seem to go wrong. You feel frustrated and overwhelmed, as if you're carrying the weight of the world on your shoulders. In that case, a trapped emotion may lodge in one of your shoulders. The reality is that any emotion can get stuck anywhere in the body.

If you don't notice the imbalance, it can go on for years. Eventually, it may cause real problems with your health, both mental and physical.

The Dual Nature of Trapped Emotions

Trapped emotions affect you in two distinct ways, mentally and physically. Let's talk about how they affect you mentally first. They will cause you to feel an exaggerated emotional response. Let's first examine some real-life situations where trapped emotions were exerting an obvious mental affect.

Marie and Her Trauma

One of the most dramatic examples of this occurred with Marie, a beautiful and kind-hearted patient in her fifties. A year before she came to me, her only son had been brutally murdered. As you might imagine, the death of her son was a horrible blow to Marie. To make matters worse, the trial of her son's murderer kept getting delayed in the courts, so she couldn't put it behind her.

She was having a difficult time dealing with life when she first came to see me. In the year since her son's murder, she'd been completely caught up in her grief and loss. When we tested her for trapped emotions, we found one after another related to her son and his death. We released them. After that, Marie was free. She went back to being the well-balanced person she always was. Even though she misses her son and will always feel his absence, she's one of the happiest, most well-balanced people I know.

Her trapped emotions were throwing her off-balance by sustaining a negative vibration. Once we eliminated them, she was able to deal with her loss in a healthier way.

Sarah and the JFK Assassination

I will never forget Sarah, a 71 year old woman who came to me for treatment. I began to ask her subconscious mind through muscle testing what she needed. We found that she had a trapped emotion of sadness.

While your conscious mind may not remember things very well, your subconscious mind remembers everything that has ever happened to you. Of course, it also knows about each trapped emotion in detail. It knows when the trapped emotion occurred, what the precise emotion was, who was involved, and more.

As I questioned Sarah's subconscious mind about this trapped emotion, I tried to determine when it had occurred. It turned out that the emotion of sadness had become trapped in Sarah's body in 1963.

On a hunch, I asked, "Is this sadness about the assassination of John F. Kennedy?" The answer her body gave through muscle testing was "Yes." The moment we arrived at this, she burst into tears. As her tears flowed, she said, "Oh, yes, that affected me so deeply. And then when President Kennedy's son, John, Jr., died in that plane crash a few years ago, it brought it all back to me. I couldn't do anything but cry for days."

If you're old enough to remember that day in November 1963, you'll recall how shocking and sad it was. On that day, Sarah's whole being was filled with sadness. The emotion was overwhelming. It was too intense to be processed by her physical body, and as a result, it became trapped.

Trapped Emotions Affect Us Emotionally

Trapped emotions generate a specific energetic vibration. They're also associated in our minds with specific kinds of events. In Sarah's case, the emotion of sadness — resonating at its own particular frequency — was specifically connected in her mindbody to the sudden death of a Kennedy. When John Kennedy Jr. was tragically killed, her natural sadness for that event was amplified by the trapped emotion already stuck inside her. Part of her body, where the energy of this emotion was lodged, was already functioning as best it could, immersed for nearly forty years in the sadness of JFK's death.

When she got the news of John Kennedy Junior's death, her entire body fell into resonance with the emotion that was trapped. The result was that, instead of crying a little and moving on, Sarah cried for days, and the pain of that day in November 1963, came back to her full-force. In fact, that pain had never really left her at all. In a literal and fascinating way, part of her body had never stopped feeling that deep sadness.

This is a perfect example of how a trapped emotion can persist for many years and cause you to experience similar emotions in an exaggerated way.

When trapped emotions are never released, you may feel that pain and heightened response for the rest of your life. It's so unnecessary, because your trapped emotions can easily be gotten rid of.

The Rest of the Story

Before I released her sadness, I decided to ask where this emotion had been residing in her body for almost four decades. What tissues in her body had been laboring within the sphere of this deep sadness all those years? What was the effect upon those tissues? The subconscious mind knows these answers full well, and finding out is as easy as asking. The answer shocked both of us.

Muscle testing showed that the trapped emotion of sadness was lodged in the area of her left breast.

Sarah and I stared at each other for a moment in wonder. She was a survivor of breast cancer. Four years before, her left breast had been removed in a surgical mastectomy.

This trapped emotional energy had become lodged in her left breast, where it remained. Why her left breast and not some other area of the body? Perhaps she had a greater vulnerability in her left breast due to a low-grade infection, a prior injury, or some other imbalance.

My own feeling is that it became trapped in these tissues — that lay so close to her heart — because of her love for President John F. Kennedy.

Whatever the reason for its location, the trapped emotion stayed in her body as the years went by. It caused a constant low-level irritation in her tissues, and this may have been a contributing factor to the cancer. The signs were not recognized soon enough, and ultimately her left breast had to be removed to save her life, but the sadness remained. Releasing that trapped sadness from her body helped her to heal emotionally. I only wish I could have discovered it years earlier, which might have helped her avoid a lot of pain and suffering, and might have even helped her avoid breast cancer.

The Physical Effects of Trapped Emotions

Tissues that are continually being distorted by a trapped emotion will eventually suffer the effects of it.

If you take a magnet and hold it close to an older tube-type television screen or computer monitor, you will see a very visible distortion of the picture. This is because the magnetic field is interfering with the normal flow of electrons within the screen. If you get the magnet too close, or if you leave the magnet there long enough, it will create a permanent distortion and even ruin the screen. Trapped emotions affect the body in a similar way. After all, the body is energy, and so are trapped emotions. But trapped emotions are a *negative* energy, and distort the body's tissues, just as the magnet distorts the picture on the TV screen. Distort the body tissues long-term, and pain and malfunction will be the result. This is why the release of a trapped emotion will often cause immediate relief of discomfort and other symptoms, and possibly the reversal of some diseases.

I think that this is very fertile ground for further research, which could yield profound insight into the disease process.

It is my experience that trapped emotions can exert an astonishing influence over the tissues of the body. What happens when those tissues are continually irritated over time? The first symptom is often pain or subtle malfunction which can be difficult to detect. If tissues are irritated over a long period of time, the tissue may eventually enter into a state of *metaplasia*, or change. In other words, the specific type of cell begins to revert back to a more primitive cell. The next step is malignancy, or cancer.

While there are a variety of things that are thought to cause cancer, I believe firmly that trapped emotions are a contributing factor to the disease process, as I believe they are to many, if not most other diseases.

Every cancer patient I treated was found to have trapped emotions embedded in the malignant tissues.

It is possible that some of these energies may have been attracted to the area precisely because the tissues were in a severe state of imbalance. While this is possible and even likely as the disease progresses, trapped emotions are, in my opinion, an underlying cause of cancer. It is vital that these trapped emotions be removed. Even though they may have already contributed to the cancer, once removed, they cannot cause any further damage in the years to come.

Rochelle's Lung Cancer

When Rochelle first came to me for treatment, she had a cancer the size of a baseball in her lung. She was going through chemotherapy when we met. I asked her body if there were trapped emotions in this malignant lung tissue and the response was "Yes."

The trapped emotions in Rochelle's tumor dated back many years, to a time when she was a young woman. She is Filipino, and had married an American sailor stationed in the Philippines. After they had a child together, Rochelle's husband was away at sea for six months or more at a time. She'd expected his frequent absences and had come to terms with the separation in her conscious mind, but raising a child by herself was difficult and lonely. Consciously, Rochelle believed she was fine with his absence. But her body revealed that the emotions of resentment, frustration and abandonment had become trapped inside of her during this period.

"No, no," Rochelle insisted. "I never felt that way. I knew Danny would be gone and it was fine with me. I was OK on my own." And yet, after I'd run the magnet down her back, Rochelle sat up and shook her head. "You know, it's the funniest thing," she said. "I feel so much lighter, like a weight has been lifted from my chest."

Since she had to drive 90 minutes each way to my clinic, I only saw Rochelle three times, but it was enough for me to release all the trapped emotions that showed up in the area of her tumor. About five weeks later, she showed up at my office ecstatic over the good news. Her doctors had taken a new x-ray and the tumor was completely gone from her lung.

Could the trapped emotions have been a significant contributing factor in the creation of this cancer? I believe that the answer is yes.

Of course, I can't prove that the release of the trapped emotions eliminated the tumor, since Rochelle was also undergoing chemotherapy. But by removing the emotions that were lodged in her chest, we may have made the chemotherapy more effective, and their removal may have given her body the edge it needed to heal. I hope to live long enough to see a day when all patients will be treated with the best of all methods like this.

Jean's Painful Ovary

One of the things about trapped emotions that surprised me the most was their ability to cause physical pain. The very first experience that I had with this phenomenon was quite dramatic. My wife, Jean suddenly began experiencing acute and severe pain in her left lower abdomen. Muscle testing showed that the pain was coming from her left ovary, and that the cause was emotional. As rapidly as I could, I began to identify the emotion responsible. To my surprise, I ended up finding not one but six different emotions. As you will learn later on, we release trapped emotions one at a time. Sometimes, more than one trapped emotion will be found nested in the same area, such as in this case. With the exception of the last emotion, all of them had to do with tragic or upsetting events that had occurred in the lives of women that were close to Jean. I released each trapped emotion as it was identified.

Amazingly, her pain level decreased instantly and noticeably with each trapped emotion that I released. After clearing five trapped emotions, her pain level was a fraction of what it had been only moments before.

Her body indicated that there was one more trapped emotion. Testing quickly revealed that an emotion of feeling *worthless* had become trapped when Jean was in kindergarten.

The year was 1960. It was an election year, and the contest was between Richard M. Nixon and John F. Kennedy. Jean's teacher informed her that a boy and a girl from the school had been chosen to be interviewed by the local newspaper about the upcoming presidential election, and that she was one of those chosen. She was told that she would be asked some questions about the candidates, particularly who she would vote for if she could.

She was excited, and the big day soon came. She was ushered into a room at the school that had been prepared for the interview. There were two chairs set up right in front, one for each child. The interviewer began asking questions of the little boy first, while flash bulbs popped as his picture was taken. Although her picture was taken, for some reason, no questions were asked of Jean at all. She was ignored almost completely, with the exception of being told how to pose for the photo. Suddenly the interview was over. As she was ushered back to her classroom she felt confused. Gradually it began to dawn on her how unimportant she must be.

She began to feel worthless, and she felt the emotion strongly enough that it became trapped in her physical body.

Emotions are energy, and the specific vibration of an emotion determines precisely which emotion it is. A trapped emotion is like a little ball of energy which will always "land" or become lodged somewhere in the physical body. For some reason, this trapped emotion of worthlessness lodged in Jean's left ovary, where it remained for thirty years.

When we released this last trapped emotion, the remnants of her pain were instantaneously gone. She got up off the floor and we looked at each other in mutual amazement at what we had just experienced. Jean has never had a recurrence of pain in that area. I can't help but wonder what the consequences to her health might have been if we had not released those energies from her ovary.

Jack's Tennis Elbow

Another example of how trapped emotions can cause physical pain came from a patient of mine named

Jack. He was 42 years old when he came to me for treatment of his excruciating tennis elbow, which he'd been suffering from for months. The discomfort in his right forearm had become so great that he could no longer even turn the key to start his car without terrible pain. I began treating him with a traditional chiropractic approach of spinal and extremity adjustments and physical therapy. After working on him for about a week, I didn't see much improvement and that surprised me. Tennis elbow is an ailment that is normally treated very successfully with chiropractic care.

I was frustrated with Jack's lack of improvement. This was in the early days of my work with trapped emotions, and I hadn't yet thought to ask his subconscious if emotions had anything to do with his problem. I was just beginning to understand how powerful trapped emotions can be, and how they can cause many different kinds of symptoms. I knew they could cause physical pain, but I also knew that tennis elbow was an inflammatory condition that I had treated successfully before. However, since I was having no results with the traditional approach, I decided to ask Jack's subconscious if trapped emotions were an underlying cause of his tennis elbow. I was a bit surprised when his body answered, "Yes."

High School Girls

Using the Emotion Code, we identified the first emotion. According to his body, the trapped emotion was *inferiority*. It had become trapped in his body during high school, and had to do with a certain girl he'd liked. I released it, and Jack was surprised by the immediate effect this had on his arm. Suddenly his elbow pain had decreased noticeably. I asked again if there were any trapped emotions that we could release. His body answered "Yes", so I began asking what the next emotion was, when it had become trapped, and if it had to do with anyone in particular. This trapped emotion was also from Jack's high school days, and was the result of a less than satisfactory relationship – with a different girl this time. The trapped emotion was *nervousness*. When we released it, Jack's elbow pain lessened even more significantly. We continued this process until we had removed a total of five trapped emotions.

They were all from high school, and each emotion involved a different girl. His wife, who was there with him during his treatment seemed amused.

As we released each trapped emotion, the discomfort level in Jack's forearm noticeably decreased. The moment we released the last emotion, his pain was completely gone! He turned his arm this way and that. He imitated turning the key in his car. There was no pain whatsoever.

He had suddenly regained his full range of motion in his elbow joint, and I could reproduce no pain by pressing my fingers into the muscles of his forearm, which previously had been very painful to the touch. This result was astounding to all of us that were witness to it.

Jack was a tennis player during high school, but hadn't picked up a racket in years. Trapped emotions tend to gravitate toward weaker areas of the body, where there is extra stress, an injury or an infection, or some other imbalance. All of these particular trapped emotions lodged in the tissues of Jack's forearm. I believe this is because during high school, his forearm was being repeatedly stressed and even injured to a degree. At the same time, he was experiencing emotional distress and picking up trapped emotions from his failing attempts at romance. Remember that a trapped emotion will always land somewhere, likely at the weakest link in the body's chain.

I still think if I hadn't been there and seen it for myself, I wouldn't believe it.

Within a matter of a few minutes, Jack's pain went from crippling to non-existent.

I was once again amazed that emotions could somehow directly cause such dramatic physical pain. Nevertheless, I had just seen it with my own eyes. As I continued to use the Emotion Code on my patients, I was amazed by how many conditions were actually being caused in whole or in part by trapped emotions, and by how destructive they were to my patients' health.

Powerful healing occurs when trapped emotions are finally released. Who knows how much pain, unhappiness and chronic illness could be completely avoided by eliminating trapped emotions! I quickly learned that some of the feelings trapped within my patients' bodies had been there for much longer than I would have thought possible. It made me sad to think that, at some level, these patients had been suffering constantly for all those years, from something that is so easy to get rid of.

Phobias

A phobia is defined as an irrational, persistent fear of certain activities, persons, objects or situations. I have found that trapped emotions are a significant cause of phobias, perhaps the only cause. The subconscious mind knows what the underlying cause of the phobia is, and each phobia has one or more trapped emotions that are the cause.

The Airplane Picture Phobia

It is possible to have a phobia about literally anything. For example, I once treated a woman who had a rather odd phobia. She could not look upon a picture of an aircraft in a magazine or see one on television without having a severe panic attack. If a jet flew overhead, she had to keep her eyes on the ground. If she looked up at the plane, she would have an attack.

I asked her subconscious mind through muscle testing if there was a trapped emotion that was causing her phobia. The answer was, "Yes." Through further testing I was able to determine what had happened.

A number of years earlier she had been reading a magazine article about the crash of a passenger jet. The article was accompanied by a photograph of the jet taken just before impact.

As she read this article, she was overcome with emotion. She identified strongly with the terrified passengers, and a trapped emotion was created. I released the emotion, and the phobia was instantly gone. She was able to look at airplanes both in photographs and in the sky immediately without any trouble, and her phobia did not return.

Night Terrors

In another case, a 42 year-old patient named Carol had suffered from night terrors nearly all her life. Her screams of terror would awaken her husband and children at least three nights every week! Night terrors differ from nightmares in that they don't seem to be caused by a specific dream. Instead, a specific and very frightening emotion is felt while the victim is asleep.

Her night terrors had been a major problem for most of her life. She had broken both collar bones, multiple ribs and had even sustained a skull fracture due to her flailing attempts to escape her terrorizing dream-state.

Her subconscious mind responded affirmatively to my simple question, "Is there a trapped emotion that is causing your night terrors?" A little further testing revealed that emotions of panic, terror and fear had become trapped in her body when she was five years old, during a short period when she was experiencing a recurring nightmare. The nightmare was long since gone, but the trapped emotions remained.

The result of releasing these trapped emotions was that within one week the night terrors were gone for good, and did not return.

Can You Afford to Keep Them?

I believe that removing trapped emotions is vital to your quality of life. Removing them may prevent many different problems from eventually occurring. Hopefully you are beginning to understand how releasing your trapped emotions can give you relief from mental and physical symptoms you may be suffering from now.

By releasing your trapped emotions, you will be removing the unwanted negative energy-clouds that are hampering the normal function of your tissues, and you will be helping to re-establish the free flow of energy, thus helping your body to heal itself.

Your mind will return to a more natural state as well, without the drama, pain and weight of your old emotions blocking you from progressing in your life.

Next, I will share some amazing secrets that ancient physicians knew about the human energy field that have just recently been rediscovered.

PART II

THE ENERGETIC WORLD

OUR BIRTH IS BUT A SLEEP AND A FORGETTING:
THE SOUL THAT RISES WITH US, OUR LIFE'S STAR,
HATH HAD ELSEWHERE ITS SETTING,
AND COMETH FROM AFAR.
NOT IN ENTIRE FORGETFULNESS,
AND NOT IN UTTER NAKEDNESS,
BUT TRAILING CLOUDS OF GLORY
DO WE COME FROM GOD,
WHO IS OUR HOME.

- WILLIAM WORDSWORTH

3

MYSTERIES OF THE
ANCIENT ENERGY HEALERS

In 1939, a Russian electrical technician named
Semyon Kirlian discovered what is now known
as Kirlian photography.[1] Kirlian photography uses
pulsed, high voltage frequencies to take pictures of the
radiating energy fields that surround all living things.
The technique is also referred to as Gas Discharge
Visualization, or GDV.

Russian scientists have performed a significant amount
of research using Kirlian photography over the last
65 years, and have found that all things exhibit the
characteristics of an energy field, although living
things have a much more vibrant energy field than

---

1 John Iovine, *Kirlian Photography: A Hands-on Guide* (Victoria, Australia: Images
Publishing, 2000), 24.

inanimate objects.[2] Perhaps the most striking Kirlian images are those of leaves which have been cut in half, yet still show the complete, intact energy fields of the whole leaves.[3] Is it possible that these Kirlian images are actually revealing the inner, spiritual nature of things?

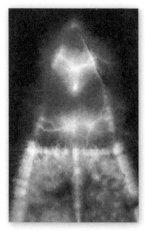

Kirlian Photo of Cut Leaf

The existence of the "Human Energy Field" has been a basic tenet of the healing arts for a very long time. The Hindus understood the vital, life-giving force which permeates and gives life to all things to be *Prana*, an understanding going back 5,000 years. The Chinese taught that this energy is called *Chi*, and understood that if the Chi is imbalanced within an individual, the result is poor health.

Throughout history, as many as 97 diverse and separate cultures had a belief in the human energy field.

Trapped emotions distort and block the flow of this energy, and the Emotion Code is one simple way to bring this energy back to a more balanced state.

---

2 Ioivine, 25

3 "Fotograferingsteknik som visar en aura runt föremålen. Uppfanns av ryssen Semyon Kirlian." <http://paranormal.se/topic/kirlianfotografi.html>

The Spirit and the Temple

I believe the human energy field is essentially the spirit that exists within each of us. I believe that if you could somehow magically pull your spirit out of your body and stand them alongside each other for comparison, the likeness would surprise you.

Many of the near-death experiences that have been recorded reveal that people who have "died" have actually just left their bodies for a time. Sometimes they don't even realize that they have died until they look down and see their physical body lying there as they hover above it. Individuals such as these have come to know by their own experience that they are not their physical body. Instead, their body is more like a temple that houses their spirit-self.

I had an experience once that I will never forget, as it taught me the truth of this concept. When I was in practice I regularly saw many patients with difficult and chronic conditions. I was in the habit of saying a short and silent prayer to God for guidance before each treatment, and I came to appreciate His help on many occasions when my own knowledge proved inadequate.

One day, after uttering a silent prayer for help, I turned my attention to the patient lying on the table before me. At that moment, I was given a gift of understanding from above. I perceived that I was standing in the presence of a sacred temple; the temple of the body. I was filled with the deepest sense of awe and reverence. This inspired perception revealed the truth about the body on a much higher level of understanding than I'd ever had before.

This spiritual experience changed how I see people. I have always had a lot of love and respect for mankind, but now I realize that the truth of our existence is more profound and sacred than we imagine. We truly are spiritual beings, having a physical experience here on this earth.

How Your Thoughts Affect Others

Your thoughts originate from your spirit intelligence and can have a profound effect on those around you. Your thoughts are energy, and are continually radiating from your body, without limits.

The energy of your thoughts and feelings exerts a subtle effect on other people as well as other forms of life. We are constantly making contact with others whether we realize it or not, since all energy is continuous and connected.

A patient named Linda came to me suffering from Chronic Fatigue Syndrome. She expressed to me that the symptoms of her illness started after she began sharing a cubicle with a very negative woman at her office. This woman was constantly seething about one thing or another. Linda felt that this woman's negative energy had triggered the downward spiral of her health.

Thoughts are Things

Ancient healers had a profound understanding of the power of thought. In my seminars I use a simple test to illustrate how thoughts can have a powerful effect on another person's mind and body, even at a distance.

I have a volunteer stand at the front of the room with his back to the audience. I perform a quick baseline muscle test to make sure he is testable, by having him say "love", and then pressing down gently but firmly on his outstretched arm. This should give a strong muscle response, and he should be able to resist my downward pressure without any trouble. Then I have him say "hate", and again I press down on his arm, which now is weakened, making him unable to resist.

After making sure we are ready for the demonstration, I instruct the volunteer to keep his eyes closed and his mind clear. I make sure to keep my mind clear as well, so I won't interfere with the demonstration. I then instruct the audience that when I give the thumbs-up signal behind his back, they are to silently send positive thoughts to the volunteer, such as "I love you", or "You are wonderful." I tell the audience that when I give the thumbs down signal behind his back, they are to think negative thoughts about the volunteer, such as "I hate you", or "You are disgusting."

At my thumbs-up signal, the audience begins sending positive thoughts toward him, and I gently push down on his outstretched arm. I remain silent during the demonstration to illustrate to everyone in the audience that it is their thought energy alone that is creating the effect. Without exception, the subject's arm is always strong.

Then I give the thumbs-down signal and the audience begins sending negative thoughts to the volunteer. I press down on his arm again, but instead of being strong, his arm is invariably weak. Remember that during this process, he is not consciously aware of what signals I am giving the audience. He not only has his back to them, but my communication with the audience is non-vocal, my hand signals to them are given behind his back, and his eyes are closed.

This simple test has given consistently reliable results during all my years of teaching seminars. It works because we are made of energy, and thoughts are energy, too. When thought energy from others passes through your energetic being, there must always be an effect, either positive or negative. In this case, the audience's negative thoughts about the volunteer weaken him demonstrably. Their positive thoughts strengthen him. This fascinating, yet simple test has some rather profound implications.

Of course, your own thoughts will have the most drastic and immediate effect on the state of your own energy field. Shifting your thinking from positive to negative will immediately shift your vibrational energy from positive to negative. This will inevitably produce negative results, the most obvious and immediate of which is a generalized weakening of the body. You might imagine how negative thoughts have a weakening affect on your body's organs and tissues, and how continuing in this state might be dangerous to your health and well-being.

Your subconscious mind is aware of negative thoughts that might be harming you, whether they are your own thoughts or not. Often your conscious mind is slow to detect negative energies if you cannot see proof of them, like facial expressions, body language or verbal communication. This "proof" is what you have been taught to look for since you were a little child.

I think we have all been somewhat desensitized, and so most of us are unable to consciously detect energy that we cannot see.

We have been bombarded with information since the day we were born about what the world is supposed to be like.

We are fed perspectives, opinions, prejudices, traditions, theories, facts, and doctrines. We hope that what we have learned is based in truth. We go to school to learn the "facts" about nature, science and the history of the world. By the time we reach adulthood, our ideas about the world are essentially in place.

When new information comes along, it is only natural that our minds are slow to accept and understand things that don't fit with previously learned information. It might be hard to accept if the new information requires us to make some changes in our thinking, especially if it goes against what we've been taught.

The Nature of Things

Most of us never learned that everything around us is made of energy, vibrating at different levels, making things look different, taste different, smell different, and feel different. We live in what I like to call a "Lego" universe. In case you have been living in a cave, (or perhaps have no experience with children) Legos are little plastic building blocks that come in various colors, shapes and sizes. Anyone who has been to a Legoland theme park can tell you that these little plastic building blocks can be used to build anything from elephants to skyscrapers.

Our universe is also made of little building blocks called subatomic particles. They are actually not particles at all, but you can think of them as infinitesimally small units of vibrating energy. If you put enough of these little energies together, you have an atom. Like Legos, differing arrangements of these little energies will produce atoms of different elements, such as hydrogen, carbon, titanium and so on. Again, like Legos, various atoms can be arranged to make molecules that we call proteins, fats, carbohydrates, and so on. Ultimately, all the things we see around us and literally everything that exists, whether plant, animal, mineral, gas, liquid, solid or anything else, is made of these little building blocks, and they are made of energy.

The Mysterious Quantum World

Subatomic particles are not really particles; they are instead a "quantum", or a quantity of something that is quite indefinable. Quantum physics, or the study of these smallest units of energy, was started by Albert Einstein and his contemporaries. These brilliant scientists devised some very ingenious experiments in an attempt to discover more about the nature of these energies. One of the most startling aspects of quantum research reveals that these energies behave in different ways depending on what the observer is expecting to see. Many physicists believe that the only explanation for these mysterious behaviors is that the energies within the atom are themselves *intelligent* to some small degree.[4]

In one famous experiment, scientists split an atom, sending two of its particles (or energies) traveling in different directions at nearly the speed of light. After the particles had journeyed a certain distance in different directions, one of the particles passed through a powerful magnetic field which changed its direction of travel. At the same instant, its sister particle changed <u>direction too-</u> at precisely the same angle. Though a

4 Jerry D. Wheatley, *The Nature of Consciousness*, (Phoenix, AZ: Research Scientific Press), 668.

considerable distance separated them, the two particles were still mysteriously connected. What happened to one instantly affected the other, with no regard to distance or separation. How do you think this could be? How could these little energies perform such a feat of apparently instantaneous communication if they were so far apart?[5]

No one really knows for certain, at least not yet. However, quantum physics has shown this phenomenon over and over again. Making a change in one particle will cause an instantaneous and equivalent change in a connected particle, no matter how far away it is. It appears that distance is no barrier to the connectedness of their energy. Remember, everything is connected to everything else![6]

Remembering the Kamikazes

This inexplicable phenomenon is not restricted to the behavior of individual subatomic particles, however. This strange connectedness has been shown to occur in the cells in the human body.

In one well-known study, white blood cells were taken from a subject and placed in a Petri dish. White blood cells are responsible for seeking out and destroying foreign bacteria, toxins, and other invaders. The subject was hooked up to electrodes to measure the electrical

5 Dr. Lee Warren, B.A., D.D., *Connectedness Part 1,*
<http://www.plim.org/Connectedness.htm>
6 P.C.W. Davies, Julian R. Brown, *The Ghost in the Atom: A Discussion of the Mysteries of Quantum Physics* (Cambridge, UK: Cambridge University Press, 1999), .

activity of his body. His white blood cells were also placed in a highly sensitive device that was able to measure their electrical activity. Exact measurements were taken of the electrical activity level of both the patient and his white cells.

One of the men in the study had served in the Navy during World War II on an aircraft carrier stationed in the Pacific. While he was there, Japanese kamikaze suicide pilots had attacked. The man was terrified, and more than once, he was sure he was going to die.

After he was hooked up to the electrodes, he was shown newsreel footage of kamikaze pilots diving and attacking aircraft carriers during the war. While it was a long-ago event, his body had not forgotten it. The sudden acute anxiety that he felt showed immediately on the readout from the electrodes on his body.

This comes as no real surprise. But the researchers were amazed to see that his white blood cells on the other side of the room showed exactly the same burst on the readout. Both readouts were essentially identical. The electrical currents of the cells were suddenly just as erratic as the currents in his body. They turned off the projector, and the electrical activity in both the man and his blood cells across the room returned to normal.

The scientists could hardly believe it. They repeated the test a number of times, with similar results each time. Just to see what would happen, the test was repeated again but the distance between the patient and his white blood cells was increased. In fact, the measuring device containing the still-living white blood cells was driven to another laboratory a number of miles away, and the test was repeated.

Keeping precise records of the times and electrical activities of the man in the room and his cells several miles away, they repeated the experiment again and again. The man was shown the kamikaze clips, then allowed to relax. Then he was shown the newsreels again and allowed to relax. The electrical activity on the man's readouts and those of his living blood cells several miles away matched every time.

The results of this test went against everything these scientists had been taught. Ask anyone whether a man who gets upset watching a movie can make his blood cells act upset – many miles away – and you'll probably be laughed at. It sounds impossible, yet it really happened.[7]

The Intelligent Universe

Other things even more amazing than this have happened as well. They seem absolutely miraculous because we don't understand them. In fact, we are just now beginning to understand the mysterious nature of energy, how it works and how it can be harnessed.

---

7 Deepak Chopra televised lecture, April 2004.

I believe that one of the greatest secrets of the universe is just now beginning to be unveiled.

This great secret has to do with the modern discovery of the intelligent nature of subatomic particles, or the intelligent nature of energy.

Imagine for a moment that what quantum physicists are saying is actually true. Imagine for a moment that the universe in which we live is entirely made of energies that are themselves somehow intelligent.

Think about this. The chair you are sitting in right now is made of energy. That energy is intelligent. Your chair can't "think", but on some level, your chair is composed of countless little energies that are doing precisely what they are supposed to do to keep your chair in one piece, helping to make your experience in this world what it is.

Max Planck, one of the greatest minds of the 20th century, considered the father of Quantum Theory, made the following statement when he was awarded the Nobel prize for physics:

As a man who has devoted his whole life to the most clear headed science, to the study of matter, I can tell you as a result of my research about atoms this much: There is no matter as such. All matter originates and exists only by virtue of a force which brings the particle of an atom to vibration and holds this most minute solar system of the atom together. We must assume behind this force the existence of a conscious and intelligent mind. This mind is the matrix of all matter.

The Power of Intention

Your intention is really just another form of energy. I like to think of it as a directed form of thought energy.

Because energy is intelligent, it actually has the ability to *obey,* or *cooperate* with your intention.

Ancient healers demonstrated an understanding of this concept, that the universe is filled with and made of intelligent energy, which is able to respond to intention.

Jesus Christ is still known as the greatest healer of all time, as he routinely healed the blind and crippled, and even raised the dead. His first miracle, though not about healing, dramatically demonstrates the concept of intelligent energy.

Jesus was with his disciples at a wedding where the host ran out of wine, a terrible faux pas in those days. Jesus directed the servants to fill some large vessels with water, which he then turned to wine to the astonishment of all those present. I believe that Jesus simply told the water to become wine, and it simply obeyed his word. But I believe it worked because the water itself was intelligent, and therefore able to obey Christ's command (John 2:1-11, KJV).

Feel Like Walking on Water?

Another example from the Bible is a story involving the apostle Peter. Jesus had sent his apostles to cross the sea while he went up on a mountain to pray. The apostles were on their ship, in the midst of a stormy sea, when in the early hours of the morning they saw a figure walking toward them on the water. The apostles were terrified, and thought it was a ghost. When they realized it was their master, Peter cried out to Him, "Lord, if it be thou, bid me come unto thee on the water." Jesus said, "Come." Peter got out of the boat and began walking on the water toward Jesus. He was walking on water! But when he looked around and realized how unnatural it was to be doing what he was doing, and how bad the storm was, he began to fear, and immediately started to sink. Peter cried out, "Lord save me!" Jesus reached out and caught him. Jesus said, "Oh thou of little faith, wherefore didst thou doubt?" (Matt 14:22-31, KJV).

Peter started out with faith, the belief that he could walk on water. His faith and intention were so powerful that he was actually able to do it. The intelligences of the water simply responded to his belief, to his intention, in a very immediate way, and the normal state of things instantly changed to support his intention. The moment Peter began to fear, his clear intention and faith in his own ability to walk on water began to diminish. As his faith diminished, his clear intention vanished, and he began to sink, because the universe had to respond to his new state of mind.

You see, Peter began to sink because he began to doubt, to fear. Doubt and fear are the opposites of faith, and they cannot coexist.

The universe supports your beliefs about yourself, too. If you think you can't, the universe will support that belief, and you will not succeed.

On the other hand, if you think you can, the universe will support that belief, and you will be empowered.

Walking on Air

About two months after the death of my father, I had a very unusual dream. It was profound to me, and I took it as a message from God. I dreamed that I was walking down a hallway in a university or a college. The hallway was filled with busy people on their own errands. There were people all around me, but there was something very unusual happening to me. I was literally walking on air, about an inch off the floor. The feeling was absolutely incredible. I tried walking faster, then slower, to see if it would change my altitude. It didn't change, I was still walking about an inch off the floor, and the feeling was indescribable!

No one around me seemed to notice this, as they were intent on what they were doing. I thought to myself, "If I can walk an inch off the ground, I'll bet I can walk a foot off the ground." As soon as I thought this, it was done! I was walking a foot off the ground! I looked behind me at that point, and saw a group of small children, whose eyes were fastened upon me. They were also walking a foot off the ground, just like me, although no one else seemed to notice what was happening.

I continued walking, and found I could gain altitude as I desired, and before long, my head was nearly touching the ceiling.

At this point, I noticed that everyone had stopped what they were doing and had turned their faces up toward me. They were questioning me, saying, "How are you doing that? How can you possibly be doing what you're doing?"

The answer I gave them was a message from God to me, and now is a message from God to you.

I said to them, "It's easy! All you have to do is *believe* you can do it, and be grateful to God that you are *doing* it!"

Then I looked further down the hallway, and saw several large glass doors that led outside. There were beautiful green rolling hills, more campus buildings, and a vast open sky. I thought to myself, "When I get beyond those doors, I will be able to fly!"

It was at that moment I awakened. Still in a dreamlike state, I realized clearly what the dream meant. The fact that I could walk on air meant that I could do whatever I believed I could do, as long as I was grateful to God that I was doing it. The children symbolized the simple, pure faith of minds unfettered by a lifetime of learned limitations. The doors had a dual meaning. They symbolized the limits that we place on ourselves in this mortal life, and they also symbolized death. Part of the message was that my father was beyond those doors, and that he could fly, with no earthly limits to his abilities.

If we express this dream in the form of a mathematical equation, it would look like this:

Your Belief That You Can Do It
+ Your Gratitude To God That You Are Doing It
= The Results You Want To Obtain

Would we ever begin anything if we did not believe we could do it? No. Belief is essential to all we do, and is the necessary first step.

Gratitude is an essential part of this equation, and I can't overemphasize the importance of the word *doing*. In other words, your gratitude to God that you are *doing* it is significant, because it is to God that we owe everything that we have and are, and it is to Him that we owe every opportunity that lies is in our path. If you have a goal that you want to achieve, imagine how grateful you would feel if you had already achieved it; if you can feel it and expect that it will be, it will be.

As you learn to cultivate gratitude to God for what you already have, your faith and belief will increase, for you will draw yourself closer to that very source of power from which all things flow.

You will soon find yourself doing the very thing that was once only a dream.

When your heart is full of gratitude, do you think it is possible to feel doubt or fear? I don't think so. To be a healer, you must not entertain thoughts of doubt; you must leave your fears behind. Your heart must be filled with love and gratitude.

Try this with the Emotion Code; it's easy. All you have to do is believe and be grateful, and you will be able to do it. I mean this very literally!

Messages from Water

A Japanese scientist, Masaru Emoto, has made a wonderful contribution to our understanding of the energetic world around us. His book, entitled The Hidden Messages in Water, details Mr. Emoto's research into the crystalline structure of water. Mr. Emoto and his colleagues found that water droplets would form widely different crystalline patterns or "snowflakes" after being exposed to different kinds of music and then frozen. Exposure to acid rock music, for example, would result in a very disrupted crystal, while a Mozart symphony would result in a beautifully formed crystal.

Taking their research further showed that by writing different words or phrases onto a piece of paper, and then taping the paper to a vial of water and leaving it overnight, different crystalline structures would result.

The phrase "I love you" would invariably result in a symmetrical, well-shaped and beautiful ice crystal, while the phrase "I hate you" would result in a very asymmetrical and disrupted crystal.

The most intensely beautiful ice crystals of all were formed when water was exposed overnight to the phrase "Love and Gratitude."[8]

Remember that your body is over 70% water. Can you see how important it is to maintain thoughts of positivity instead of negativity? Imagine how your life would be if you filled yourself with thoughts of love and gratitude on a continual basis. Imagine how people would be drawn to you. Imagine what your life could be like. I believe this is how our lives are actually intended to be!

I have read many experiences written by people who died and went to the "other side", temporarily. I have noticed that in their near-death experiences, these people were never asked what kind of car they drove

8 Masaru Emoto, David A. Thayne, *The Hidden Messages in Water*, (Hillsboro, OR: Beyond Words Publishing, Inc., 2001) 64.

on earth, or how big their bank account was. Instead, they are very often asked "How much love were you able to develop for your fellow beings?" and "How much knowledge were you able to gain on earth?"

Life is about having joy. It's about increasing our ability to give and receive love and it's about gaining all the knowledge we can. It's also about serving others, feeling grateful for all we have, and learning to create the life we want.

Trapped emotions make it more difficult for us to experience these joys and tend to short-circuit us both physically and emotionally.

The Human Energy Field

A few decades ago, scientific thought denied the existence of any sort of human energy field. Since that time, scientists have completely changed their minds. They now know with absolute certainty that an energy field exists. As new technology has come along, they've been able to test it and find out for certain. For example, one device, called the SQUID magnetometer, can detect the tiny magnetic fields created by the biochemical and physiological activities of the body.

Using this device, scientists have learned that all of the tissues and organs in the body produce specific, magnetic vibrations. They call them biomagnetic fields.[9] This is fairly new information, not widespread knowledge yet.

Although not all medical doctors are aware of this, it has been determined that the biomagnetic fields in the space around the body give a more accurate reading of the patient's health than traditional electrical measurements, like EEG's and EKG's.

In fact, scientists now know that the heart's electromagnetic field is so powerful that you can take an accurate EKG reading three feet away from the body.

The reading can be taken from any point on the body and any point in the electromagnetic field, because the field itself contains the information in a three-dimensional, or holographic way.[10]

Today's doctors know what they were taught by their professors, who learned from their professors before them, and so on. Western medicine is empirical. It's based on observation. If something can't be observed, it can't be verified. If it can't be verified, then it isn't true.

Despite its drawbacks, doctors who follow the model of western medicine have often been behind some of the most brilliant medical advances in history. They

---

9 Walter Lubeck, Frank Petter, William Rand, *The Spirit of Reiki*, (Twin Lakes, WI, Lotus Press, 2001), 72.
10 Doc Lew Childre, Howard Martin and Donna Beech, *The HeartMath Solution*, (New York, NY: Harper Collins Publishers, Inc. 1999) 260.

excel at developing important methods of precision testing, breakthrough surgical procedures and advanced technology. This model has tremendous assets, but it has its disadvantages as well.

As far back as the 1940's, Dr. Harold Saxon Burr, a distinguished medical researcher at Yale, insisted that pathology could be detected in the energy field of the body long before physical symptoms began to emerge. Although he didn't have the skills or techniques to do it himself, Burr proposed that diseases could be prevented by adjusting or manipulating the energy field.[11] His medical colleagues thought his ideas seemed unlikely and farfetched, probably because they were not taught that this could be a possibility when they were in medical school.

The importance of the energy field is still not taken into account in traditional Western medical practices, and thus, the patient often suffers needlessly due to lack of proper attention to the underlying causes of their illness.

Recently, however, many non-traditional healing practices have gone from being ridiculed to being respected. This is partially because technology has improved and scientists have been able to test more accurately, and partially because these alternative healing methods actually do work.

---

11 Robert C. Fulford, D.O., *Touch of Life: Aligning Body, Mind, and Spirit to Honor the Healer Within* (New York, NY: Pocket Books, 1996) 25.

Now mainstream science is even beginning to acknowledge the existence of the energy meridians used by ancient Chinese medical doctors for thousands of years. Acupuncture in particular is being recognized for its energetic healing power, even if it is not fully understood by the medical community. Chiropractic adjustments, which remove nerve interference, are also being proven in clinical trials to have long-lasting and significant benefits, something that chiropractic doctors and patients have known for over 100 years.

Abundant evidence exists to prove that the human body is an energetic, vibrant, emotional, and spiritual entity. The old mechanistic approach proves to be more and more limited and simplistic as we learn about the nature of energy and of the universe, and how everything is in constant communication with everything else. As Simon Mitchell points out in his book, <u>Don't Get Cancer</u>:

> A philosophy of medicine that is over-reliant on logic and limited mainly to drugs and surgery is fundamentally flawed. Acts of logic always rely on analysis, that is, breaking down a 'whole' into its constituent parts, and examining each minutely. Reductionist approaches fail to see the connectivity and relatedness of all things. As a result this philosophy is offering us 'cures' which are often as dangerous and destructive as the disease itself.

Today, we are at a turning point in medical history. With the discoveries of quantum physics and molecular biology proving that everything is energy and that it is all related, a door has been opened.

Scientific research is constantly being conducted, and continues to confirm over and over again that we are beings of energy, and that there is an intelligent force at work in the universe.

Research will continue to push back the boundaries on what we know about the human energy field. As it does so, I am convinced that the energetic basis of human thought will become more clearly understood, and that the phenomenon of trapped emotions will eventually be recognized by the scientific community for the damage they cause.

As technology continues to advance, scientists and doctors will inevitably realize how important it is to keep the body in a state of balance. The magnetic and energetic healing techniques that alternative practitioners already use will hopefully be integrated into conventional medicine to provide the best, most thorough, and most gentle healing. There is much to be learned by studying the energy of the human body, and we are the ones to gain from it. Remember that not so long ago, scientists didn't recognize that the human body had an energy field, much less that our very health depended on it!

All methods of healing are valid and have their place. In the future, I see a world where the best of all possible approaches will combine to the benefit of mankind.

Quick Fixes

I saw first-hand during my years in practice that the body has a built-in ability to heal itself, another evidence of the body's innate intelligence. The body sometimes needs help to restore itself to a state of balance. This help may consist of removing trapped emotions, detoxification, receiving chiropractic adjustments and proper nutrition, and more. Healing is a process, and it takes time.

But waiting for the body to heal itself naturally can try our patience. We usually want a quick fix. We don't want to wait; we want it now. We are conditioned by endless advertising to think that if we take a pill our problem will be solved. While some prescription medications do address the cause of illness, most only cover up the symptoms. They usually do such a wonderful job at masking our symptoms that we may think our problem is gone, when it is merely being chemically suppressed.

Remember that symptoms are the body's way of telling you that something is wrong. They are a warning signal that you need to change something, or that your body needs some help.

Masking symptoms with medications can be a bit like putting a piece of duct tape over that annoying oil light in your car that turned on recently. You may cover it up for awhile, but eventually your car will stop running.

The pharmaceutical companies would have you believe that the best way to get well is to take their products. For example, heavy advertising in the media helped to create a tremendous market for anti-depressants. While they have helped some people, like all drugs, they have side-effects. In fact, read this excerpt from an official FDA press release, dated October 14, 2004:[12]

> The Food and Drug Administration (FDA) today issued a Public Health Advisory announcing a multi-pronged strategy to warn the public about the increased risk of suicidal thoughts and behavior ("suicidality") in children and adolescents being treated with antidepressant medications…

The release of trapped emotions have consistently helped patients to overcome depression. Read this testimonial from a former patient of mine who was suffering from severe depression.

> *I had gotten to the point where I was exceedingly suicidal. Everyday I would wake up and have to decide, 'Do I live or die today?' I was stuck because part of my belief system was that my life was not mine to take. That had been a mantra already for several years, and yet I no longer wanted to live. And I happened to show up at one of Dr. Nelson's seminars where he talks about emotions. And at*

12 "FDA Launches a Multi-Pronged Strategy to Strengthen Safeguards for Children Treated With Antidepressant Medications," Oct. 15, 2004
<http://www.fda.gov/bbs/topics/news/2004/new01124.html>

that time he didn't talk about them a whole lot, and I spoke to him after he was finished speaking, and said 'You mentioned the emotions but you didn't do anything or talk about it; I need help... I don't want to live, yet I know that there are some people in this life who are happy, and there are people in this life who are functioning very well. I'm not, and I want to be. Can you do something?' And in that moment he cleared something regarding my lack of joy, and I could literally feel in the moment that he did that, all of this energy coming back to me. I actually did not sleep almost the whole night; I was so pumped and so energized after that. Since then, we have done a lot of work, mostly in the clearing of trapped emotions, and other work as well, but this emotional work is so powerful and so key. I am a different person than I was a year and a half ago. I no longer have the panic attacks; I no longer have the night terrors I used to have. I am a different person. I'm alive, I embrace life, and I love life. Thanks - Karen B.

If we have pain, we may need pain medication to be able to deal with it. I'm grateful we have it, and as I said before, all healing approaches are valid. Medications can be perfectly appropriate in the short-term, as they work to relieve symptoms, but they sometimes do more harm than good.

Witness the following article from USA Today, dated December 20, 2006:

Non-prescription pain relievers used by millions of U.S. consumers need stronger health warnings regarding liver or stomach risk, the Food and Drug Administration said Tuesday.

The drugs include some of the most commonly taken in the USA — aspirin, ibuprofen and acetaminophen — and will affect such household brands as Motrin, Advil, Aleve and Tylenol.

The FDA proposes that:

Products with acetaminophen, such as Tylenol, include warnings for liver toxicity, particularly when used in high doses, with other acetaminophen products or with three or more drinks of alcohol a day.

Over-the-counter NSAIDs (short for non-steroidal anti-inflammatory drugs) include warnings for stomach bleeding in people over 60; those who have had ulcers, take a blood thinner or more than one NSAID; or those who take them with alcohol or longer than directed.

Attention focused on their risks in 2004 when prescription NSAID Vioxx was withdrawn because of heart attack and stroke risk. Last year, the FDA sought a warning on prescription NSAID Celebrex for cardiovascular and stomach risks. An FDA advisory panel in 2002 said over-the-counter NSAIDs should have stronger warnings about stomach bleeding.[13]

---

13 Julie Schmit, Julie Appleby, "FDA calls for pain reliever warning", USA Today 20 Dec. 2006, national ed.: A.1.

Here is another testimonial from a former patient who suffered from chronic pain for four years after falling 2 stories onto a boulder and breaking her back:

I consulted Dr. Nelson because I had broken my back a few years back and had never gotten over the pain despite several types of physical therapy and exercise programs. During my first adjustment, I realized that Dr. Nelson was a true healer; I could just feel it. Almost all of my adjustments included "emotional releases" from energy blockages in my body, (unresolved traumatic events live in the energy system of the body and cause blockages in the energy flow). At first I did not notice any change, but gradually my pain began to decrease! With Dr. Nelson's help I discovered that emotions very deep within me were causing the majority of my pain... My body had so much pain stored inside from so very long ago, and Dr. Nelson was able to "talk" to my body to help me release it. What a remarkable process to experience each appointment's release and the corresponding decrease in pain. Today for the first time in 4 years I am able to work part-time, but most important of all, I feel a great healing in my physical and emotional body and have learned the invaluable fact of how these two are so integrally related. Thank you, Dr. Nelson!!!

In love and light - Linda P.

Getting to the Cause

If the essential cause of your illness is not dealt with, you will have the illness until your body is able to heal itself. I have seen many cases where the patient was on medication for their problem for years, and as soon as they went off the medication, their problem came back full swing because the underlying cause was still creating the illness. The underlying cause must be reversed or your problem will not go away and you must either remain in pain or on drugs forever.

Most of us never learned that we could access the energy of our bodies, to learn what is wrong and how to fix it. But we live in a remarkable time, when knowledge of all the ages is being poured out upon mankind beyond measure.

Ancient healing philosophies were full of truth and deep insights into our energetic nature, and the validity of these approaches is now being recognized once again.

Magnets are one of the most ancient healing modalities on earth, and are an integral part of the Emotion Code. Find out why in the next chapter.

A MAN WHO IS SWAYED BY NEGATIVE EMOTIONS MAY
HAVE GOOD ENOUGH INTENTIONS, MAY BE TRUTHFUL
IN WORD, BUT HE WILL NEVER FIND THE TRUTH.

- GHANDI

4

HEALING WITH MAGNETS

What is the most powerful healing tool in your home? Some vitamins? A prescription medication? A healing herbal tea? Something in your fridge? How about something *on* your fridge? No, not your shopping list, I'm talking about the magnet that's holding your shopping list to your fridge.

Believe it or not, the common refrigerator magnet can be one of the most powerful healing tools you'll ever own, when it comes to removing trapped emotions, provided you know how to use it. I'll explain why in this chapter.

How healthy you are is directly related to how balanced your energy field is. Energy healing works to restore and maintain the harmony of the energy field, so that the body can remain vitally healthy. But how do you begin to heal the energy field of the body if you cannot see it? You already know you can find imbalances like trapped emotions by using the Sway Test to ask the subconscious mind what is wrong. What can you use as a tool to remove trapped emotions?

The answer is you must use some other form of energy. The easiest to use, the cheapest and the most widely available energy tool is the magnet. Magnets emit pure energy and are a powerful tool to fix energetic imbalances that you cannot see.

I have used all kinds of magnets, from the most expensive and most powerful, to the least expensive and weakest. Some magnets are specifically designed for healing the body, and some are not. But I have found that virtually any magnet can be used to release trapped emotions using the Emotion Code.

Your Magnetic Existence

Your existence stretches farther than you can see or feel, precisely because you are an energetic being, even though you are also physical. It makes sense to say that if part of your existence is invisible to you, then perhaps some of the underlying causes of your health problems might be invisible to you as well.

Most people assume that they exist only inside the limits of their own skin. Your skin represents the outer layer of what you can see, and you have been taught that what you see is what is real. Now we have scientific proof that there is more to you than meets the eye.

For instance, we now know that you generate an electromagnetic field, created by the electrical activity in your body. It is created by electrical currents in your nervous system as well as the electrochemical processes that are constantly occurring in all of your cells.

Scientists now know that the electromagnetic field of your heart extends 8 to 12 feet from your body in all directions, behind you, above you, below you, in front of you and to your sides.[1]

In 1956, Japanese scientists did the groundbreaking research that proved beyond a doubt that there were both electric and magnetic forces in the body. By exposing the body to pulsing electromagnetic fields, they created electrical changes on a cellular level and altered cell metabolism. This phenomenon is known in medical science as the piezoelectric effect.

Western medicine acknowledges and accepts the existence of this electromagnetic field without reservation, but for many years has only measured the electrical component of it. Scientists and doctors have measured the body's electrical activity under clinical conditions for many years. The EKG, or electrocardiogram, which measures the electrical

---

1 Doc Lew Childre, Howard Martin and Donna Beech, *The HeartMath Solution*, (New York, NY: Harper Collins Publishers, Inc. 1999) 34..

impulses of the heart, was first put to practical use in 1895. The EEG, or electroencephalogram, which measures the electrical activity of the brain, has been used since 1913.

A basic law of physics states that whenever electrical activity is generated, a corresponding magnetic field will always occur. Scientists can measure this magnetic field using *magneto*encephalographs and *magneto*cardiograms. These machines represent a leap ahead over the old technology, which was limited to measuring only the electrical fields of the heart and brain. Scientists are coming to recognize how powerful and important these magnetic interactions are.

The brain's pineal gland, which secretes hormones that affect your whole body, is surrounded by magnetite clusters that are carefully tuned to perceive and interact with magnetic fields. These are the same kinds of magnetic clusters that allow homing pigeons, butterflies and bees to navigate using the earth's magnetic field. It appears that these magnetite formations in our own pineal glands have a lot to do with our own sense of direction. A study published in the respected British Medical Journal found that people who were suffering from calcification, or hardening of the pineal gland were significantly more likely to get lost![2]

---

2 British Medical Journal (Clin Res Ed). 1985 Dec. 21-28;291(6511):1758-9.

Floating Frogs With Magnetic Energy

Scientists attempting to understand why magnetism has such a profound affect on physiology have performed a fascinating experiment using an extremely powerful magnet and a frog. This is somewhat whimsical, but I include it because it illustrates the fact that magnets do have a physical effect.

April 12, 1997

"Scientists Make a Frog Levitate"

LONDON (AP) - British and Dutch scientists say they have succeeded in floating a frog in air -- using a magnetic field a million times stronger than that of the Earth.

And, they say, there is no reason why larger creatures, even humans shouldn't perform the same gravity defying feat.

'It's perfectly feasible if you have a large enough magnetic field,' said Peter Main, professor of physics at Nottingham University, one of the British scientists who collaborated with colleagues at the University of Nijmegen to create the first levitating amphibian.

Their endeavors are reported briefly in the current issue of the British magazine <u>New Scientist</u>.

To hold up the frog, the field had to be a million times that of the Earth, the scientists said, only then was it strong enough to distort the orbits of electrons in the frog's atoms.

'If the magnetic field pushes the frog away with sufficient force, you will overcome gravity and the frog will float,' Main said. The trick doesn't only work on frogs. Scientists say they have made plants, grasshoppers and fish float in the same way. 'Every ordinary object, whether it be a frog, a grasshopper or a sandwich, is magnetic, but it's very rare to see such a spectacular demonstration of this,' said Main.

The scientists said their frog showed no signs of distress after floating in the air inside a magnetic cylinder.[3]

Magnets and Healing

When the human body is exposed to a magnetic field, even more interesting and often surprising things happen. People's illnesses and imbalances have completely disappeared. Pain has diminished, vertigo has vanished, and fatigue has been reversed. There have been thousands of people who have had their health restored by the healing powers of magnets. Even though the proof is there, modern allopathic medicine is still currently in the experimental phase with magnets as healing tools. Many vitalistic healers already know that magnets work wonders, but medicine cannot scientifically explain the discoveries that their <u>experiments</u> have revealed.

3 "Scientists Make a Frog Levitate," *New Scientist Magazine*, 12 April 1997, 13.

In March of 2005, Time magazine ran a story about doctors at Columbia University who accidentally discovered a surprising way to cure depression – by using magnetic energy.

A Connecticut woman named Martha had been depressed for almost twenty years. She had gone through all of the recognized traditional treatments – seeing psychiatrists and psychologists, consuming any medication they gave her. But none of the treatments helped her depression. Martha decided to participate in the experimental treatment procedure at Columbia. Doctors applied a series of magnetic pulses to the top of her head. They called the treatment repetitive transcranial magnetic stimulation (rTMS).

After undergoing the hour-long procedure five times a week for six weeks, Martha said, "I started to see signs of change by about the third week. By September, I was on top again. I could take pleasure in things like food and sunshine." At the time the article came out, Martha had been returning to the institute for repeat sessions on a periodic basis, and had been depression-free for six months.

These doctors cannot explain exactly why magnetic stimulation works to cure depression and other disorders. According to Dr. George Wittenberg, a neurologist at Wake Forest University, "Magnetic stimulation is a clever way to induce current without actually having an electrical connection." The National Institute of Mental Health (NIMH) agrees that there is no denying the effectiveness of the technique, and they are sponsoring a study at Columbia and three other institutions to further test the healing effects of magnetic stimulation.[4]

In a study published in 2002 in the respected Journal of Neuropsychiatry and Clinical Neurosciences, seventy-five percent of patients suffering from depression experienced significant improvement after undergoing this same type of magnetic treatment.[5]

My Introduction to Magnets

My own exposure to the power of magnetic therapy came many years ago through my brother Greg, who had been using magnetic treatments in his chiropractic office. Greg was so enthusiastic about the effectiveness of the magnets made by a Japanese wellness company, that he finally persuaded me to give them a try in my own clinic.

The moment after I received my new magnet in the mail I found a patient that would present a real challenge. Laura had come to me for treatment of her Fibromyalgia, a debilitating condition characterized by widespread muscular pain of unknown origin. Most of Laura's pain was in her upper body. Her overall range of motion with both of her arms was very limited and

---

4 Psychiatry Res. 2004 Apr. 30;126(2):123-33.

5 Rosenberg P.B., et al. "Repetitive transcranial magnetic stimulation treatment of comorbid post traumatic stress disorder and major depression." *Journal of Neuropsychiatry and Clinical Neurosciences,* 2002 Summer;14(3):270-6.

she could barely raise them to a horizontal position without being stopped by the pain.

I explained to Laura that I'd like to try a new treatment to see what effect, if any, it might have on her condition. She agreed, and we chatted while I rolled the magnet continuously back and forth on her left arm between her shoulder and her elbow.

After a few minutes of this, I tested the range of motion in her arms again. I had her raise her right arm first, the arm we did not apply the magnet to. Laura raised her arm until it was almost horizontal to the floor. I could see that she was in pain, so I had her stop. This was what I had expected.

Then I asked her to raise her left arm, the one we had used the magnet on. To our mutual surprise, Laura raised her left arm easily and smoothly up along the side of her head without any discomfort.

Her eyes widened and she exclaimed, "I don't have any pain at all where you used that! What is that thing? Can I buy it from you?"

I put Laura through more range-of-motion tests, and to my amazement, she now had full range of motion in her left arm, and no pain. I looked down at the little silver and blue magnet in my hand with eyes as wide as Laura's. These sudden and dramatic results were quite unexpected. I told Laura all I knew, that it was a magnet designed for reducing discomfort in the body.

It took Laura very little effort to remove the cause of her symptoms. My hunch is that in her case, the biggest underlying cause of her Fibromyalgia was something that the Japanese call "MFDS", or magnetic field deficiency syndrome. Proponents of MFDS believe that you can become "deficient" in magnetic energy, just as you can become deficient in a vitamin or a mineral. Adding a little more magnetic energy to her body was all that Laura seemed to need to get rid of her pain. The relief of Laura's Fibromyalgia was just the first miracle I saw with magnets.

I believe that MFDS is a component of many illnesses. Like most illnesses, Fibromyalgia has a variety of underlying causes that can vary from person to person, and MFDS is often one of those components. In cases where it is the major or only underlying cause of the illness, the application of magnetic energy can result in dramatic improvement, as was the case with Laura.

A New Healing Tool

It was easy to put these magnets to the test, since I had a never-ending stream of people who were suffering. Sometimes the results were inexplicable and even a bit mysterious. One patient, for example, had a long-term shoulder problem that instantly went away when she put magnetic insoles in her shoes. On four separate occasions I was able to stop acute asthma attacks by simply placing a magnetic pad on the patients' chests. I saw allergies improve quickly and dramatically by placing a magnet on the surface of a patient's body. I saw bruises disappear, literally overnight. I saw broken bones heal in half the normal time.

In many cases, I came to require certain patients to wear magnets as part of their treatment protocol, because they seemed to shorten the recovery time so dramatically.

One patient had a very large disc bulge (8mm). She refused to have the recommended surgery. By the time I met her she had lost all feeling in her right leg due to nerve compression. Twenty-four hours after starting to wear a magnet over her disc injury, she began feeling sharp, shooting pains in her previously numb leg as the healing process began. Within a week she was able to stop taking all her pain medication. She continued to wear the magnet on her back, and the pain and inflammation continued to diminish and completely disappeared. One year later, her radiologist was baffled when he could find no evidence of her disc bulge upon performing a repeat CT Scan.

It's important to note that all of these cases involved the use of magnets which were specifically designed for use on the body to relieve discomfort and promote healing. (for more information see page)

Cartilage Made New

One of the most amazing healing experiences I have witnessed happened to my uncle Lovell. When he was a young man in 1937, Lovell injured his right knee. His doctors recommended surgery, but could not guarantee that the operation would help him. He decided to not have the surgery, since the odds of success and failure were about the same. As long as I knew my uncle he always had his right knee wrapped with Ace bandages. I found out later that his knee continually bothered him and caused him pain from this old injury. In 1995, a friend introduced him to magnetic therapy. This friend insisted that Lovell should put a pair of magnets on his knee for at least 10 days. These mini-magnets were about the size of a silver dollar. Lovell was skeptical, but decided that he had nothing to lose by giving it a try.

He didn't really feel any difference in his knee after five days. Even after seven days, there was no change. Finally on the tenth day something dramatic happened. To his astonishment, for the first time in 60 years he could feel no pain in his right knee. He was ecstatic and could hardly believe it. He continued to wear the magnet day and night for the next two months. His pain did not come back. At that point, he decided to have X-rays taken of his knee, so he could compare them to a previous set of X-rays that had been taken three years earlier. The old X-rays showed that the cartilage in his knee joint was almost completely gone, and the bone ends were actually touching.

To his doctor's astonishment, this new set of X-rays showed that the cartilage in his knee had somehow *regenerated*.

Although spontaneous regeneration of cartilage such as this is considered a medical impossibility, it happened.

The More We Know...

These incredible successes involving magnets forced me to open my mind to a new way of thinking – to something I'd never been taught before. But I knew I was in good company.

Most of the progress in the history of medicine has been based on creative leaps of imagination. When new treatments and methods are discovered, the old ones are abandoned to make way for a more effective style of healing. This is often a long and arduous process, since we have no guide to help us along the way, only trial and error.

As human beings, we have had our bodies for thousands of years, but since they came with no "manual", we have spent much of our time trying to figure out how they work and how to make them work better.

In former times, people thought that illness was caused by, among other things, blood that had "gone bad." As a result, bloodletting was a popular practice from antiquity until the late 1800s, until it was finally abandoned in favor of more advanced procedures.

Approved medical practices, done with the best intentions, are routinely abandoned when new insights about the body are discovered.

When I was a child, for instance, tonsillectomy or the removal of the tonsils, was considered a harmless surgery. According to one study, up to forty percent of young men entering military service in 1960 had had their tonsils removed.[6]

Back then it was believed that the tonsils were expendable, and no one really knew what they were for. Eventually, it was realized that the tonsils form an important part of the body's immune system. Today doctors are much more reluctant to take them out. This is a sign of progress in medicine.

The more we know about the true nature of the human body, the better decisions we can make involving health. While some of the healing practices from the past are not correct and have fallen by the wayside, many ancient healing methods and ideas have been right all along and are now coming back into favor.

Magnifying Your Intention

Because you are made of energy, true healing must address this aspect of your makeup. Because trapped

---

6 Robert Chamovitz, Charles H. Rammelkamp Jr., Lewis W. Wannamaker, and Floyd W. Denny Jr., "The Effect of Tonsillectomy on the Incidence of Streptococcal Respiratory Disease and its Complications," *Pediatrics* Vol. 26 No. 3 September 1960, pp. 355-367.

emotions themselves are also energy, the most efficient way to release them is with another form of energy.

Intention is a powerful form of thought-energy. It is possible to release trapped emotions using the power of your intention alone. I believe that the intention to release the trapped emotion is really the most important part of the equation.

I use magnets because I believe they literally magnify the power of your intention to get the job done.

Just as a magnifying glass magnifies an image, I believe that a magnet can literally magnify your thought-energy and intention beyond your current capacity.

This makes it possible for anyone to release trapped emotions. You don't have to be a talented or experienced healer to do this work.

If your intention is clear, using a simple magnet to magnify your intention is all you will need to achieve results formerly available only to those with vast experience.

A simple magnet can powerfully enhance the energy of your intention, and carry it into the energy field of the body. The acupuncture system provides the perfect avenue to put the energy of your intention into the body, and release the trapped emotion.

How Acupuncture Fits In

The practice of acupuncture is based on the existence of the human energy field, and has been around for thousands of years. In fact, acupuncture points (or acupoints) and meridians are described in the world's oldest known book on medicine, the Chinese <u>Huang Ti Nei-Ching</u>, or <u>The Yellow Emperor's Classic of Internal Medicine</u>, written around 2500 B.C..

Acupoints are specific locations that lie along pathways known as meridians. Meridians can be thought of as small rivers of energy that flow just beneath the skin. They follow very precise tracks over the surface of the body that do not vary from person to person.

The existence of these meridians was the subject of speculation and disagreement for many years. But in the last three decades multiple research studies have proven their existence. In one study, researcher Jean-Claude Darras injected a radioactive isotope called technetium99 into acupoints and non-acupoints alike. Radioactive isotopes such as this emit low-level radiation that can be accurately measured and mapped. The radioactive isotopes that were injected into the acupoints diffused away from them in very precise patterns that were exactly the same as the acupuncture meridians that had been mapped out anciently by Chinese physicians. The same radioactive material that had been injected into non-acupoints diffused away in no particular pattern.[7]

The Governing Meridian

Certain meridians are actually thought to function as reservoirs of energy, which connect with and supply all other acupuncture meridians. Perhaps the most important of these reservoir meridians is the Governing Meridian, which begins in the center of the upper lip, runs up and over the head, and all the way down the center of the spine, ending at the tailbone.

Because of the interconnections between the Governing Meridian and all other meridians, it provides the most

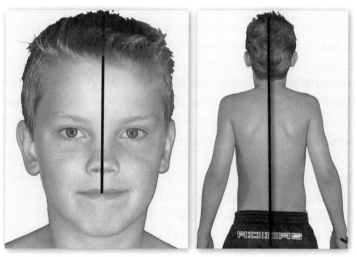

The Governing Meridian

---

7 *Journal of Nuclear Medicine*. 1992 Mar;33(3):409-12.

ideal pathway for what we want to do as we treat the body for trapped emotions using the Emotion Code. A trapped emotion is energy. To get rid of a trapped emotion, we need to overcome it with another form of energy. The Governing Meridian provides the perfect window into the body for this purpose.

Remember that a magnet actually *magnifies* your thought, which is energy. While holding the intention in your mind to release the trapped emotion that you have found, you simply pass a magnet over the Governing Meridian. Your magnified intention to release the trapped emotion enters into the Governing Meridian, and from there this thought-energy flows quickly into all the other meridians and areas of the body.

This sudden influx of intention-energy has the effect of releasing the trapped emotion permanently.

In many years of practice and many years of teaching the Emotion Code to students in seminars, we have never seen a trapped emotion return. Once you release a trapped emotion, it is gone for good.

You don't need to know any acupuncture points. You don't need to understand how it all works, really. All you need to do is have a little bit of belief and intention, and it will work. On the other hand, having some understanding of the mechanism behind it all will increase your ability as it will increase your faith in the process.

Where Does the Trapped Emotion Go?

To understand how a trapped emotion is released from the body, allow me to make an analogy. A number of companies now make special headphones that are able to cancel out background noise. These headphones can make jobs like leaf-blowing and construction work much more comfortable because they cancel out the loud noises of the machines used. Another popular use of noise-canceling headphones is for airline pilots, as the continual whine of an aircraft engine has been shown to be very fatiguing. Noise-canceling headphones sense the frequency of sound waves coming in from outside, and instantly generate a sound wave that is exactly opposite in phase. When the two sound waves collide, they cancel each other out. The result is a much quieter experience.

I believe that releasing trapped emotions may make use of a similar phenomenon. Each trapped emotion has its own particular rate of vibration, its own frequency. Just as an opposite sound wave can cancel out an extraneous noise, the energy of your magnified intention can cancel out the "noise" of a trapped emotion. When you pass a magnet over the Governing Meridian, you effectively create a flow of opposing energy in the form of magnified intention. Therefore, the trapped emotion gets cancelled out, it dissipates and disappears, similar to the noise from the jet engine.

Another example that you are perhaps more familiar with has to do with credit cards. The magnetic strip on the back of a credit card is encoded with specific information. When you place a magnet on it, you might erase the encoded information, destroying the usefulness of the credit card. Releasing a trapped emotion is similar in that the encoded emotional energy is quickly, easily and permanently erased when you swipe a magnet down the Governing Meridian.

Magnets are generally considered quite safe, but there are a few occasions when they should not be used, or should only be used after approval by a physician. These include pregnancy, use of implanted pain or insulin pumps, cochlear implants and pacemakers.

Conclusion

Begin to think of yourself as a being made of pure energy. I cannot emphasize enough how much damage trapped emotions can do. Remember that they can affect you physically, emotionally and mentally. They are made of pure energy, but they are negative energy, and the sooner you get rid of them, the better off you will be.

A simple refrigerator magnet, which you probably already own, will work to release trapped emotions.

As your intention, your clarity and your level of faith and belief in your own ability increases, you will find that the use of a magnet is optional for you. After all, your own hand is a magnetic instrument, and you always have it with you! Remember, you have a magnetic field; you are a magnetic being yourself.

You are now gaining the understanding and the power to literally become a healer by releasing trapped emotions using the Emotion Code. You will soon learn this simple procedure, which is incredibly effective and can be life-changing. The next step is to learn more ways to tap into the subconscious mind and get concrete answers.

PART III

USING THE EMOTION CODE

IS THE HUMAN BRAIN, AT SOME PRIMAL LEVEL
A WONDROUS COMPUTER LINKED WITH A
UNIVERSAL ENERGY FIELD, THAT KNOWS FAR
MORE THAN IT KNOWS IT KNOWS?

- E. WHALEN

5

GETTING ANSWERS FROM THE INNER MIND

In chapter two, you learned to use the Sway Test to connect with your subconscious mind. For some people, the Sway Test works so well and is so easily learned that it becomes the only testing method that they employ, and there is nothing wrong with that. But in this chapter, you will learn a number of other methods of testing, so you can have a variety from which to choose.

Muscle Testing

The most widely used and accepted method of accessing the internal computer system of the body is known variously as muscle testing, kinesthetic testing, or simply as kinesiology.

Although some people have never heard of it, muscle testing is not new. Doctors have been using it since the 1940s to evaluate muscle strength and assess the extent of an injury. Today physicians and others who specialize in the mechanics of body movement know that muscle testing has many more applications than doctors first believed. People are sometimes skeptical about whether it will work, but once they've seen the results for themselves, they can't help but be amazed.

Muscle testing can tell us about the overall health and balance of our bodies.

It can help identify vulnerable areas before sickness and disease take hold. It gives us a direct way to ask the body what's bothering it and, once we've treated the problem, it can tell us whether we've corrected the problem or not. It can tell us if trapped emotions are present in the body and let us know the moment they've been released. So it's no wonder that people are astounded when they see how well it works.

Holly and Her Near-Drowning

To illustrate this, let me share with you a letter I received a number of years ago from a young woman named Holly. Her Aunt Gwen has been one of my students for many years and uses muscle testing very effectively to release trapped emotions. When she was first learning the Emotion Code, she practiced it on Holly.

My Aunt Gwen came to Utah in the summer of 1999, praising a new technique she had learned. By using muscle testing, she was able to ask the body questions regarding emotions that had become 'trapped' in the body, and the body would respond to the yes or no questions effectively. She wanted to help as many people as she could with this new method, and to become proficient in the technique. I grudgingly agreed to be one of her 'victims.'

I recall standing in the room with my arm outstretched, thinking, 'This is so-o-o-o hokey!'

Then my aunt found the first trapped emotion in me: Terror.

I shrugged my shoulders. 'I don't have anything to be terrified of...'

'Shall we ask what age it comes from?' Aunt Gwen asked.

Again I shrugged my shoulders. 'Sure. I guess.'

She questioned my body, and my arm seemed to strengthen or weaken depending on what she was asking me. My arm was strong when she asked my body if this happened when I was around four years old.

'Does anything come to mind from that age?' she asked.

Immediately, I recalled my tiny, helpless fingers sliding from a metal railing and my body slipping into water above my head. My sister came and rescued me and I remembered clinging to her and repeating 'Thank you! Thank you!' over and over again.

'Yeah... I said,' reluctantly. 'I almost drowned when I was four years old.'

Aunt Gwen checked to see if this was the source of my terror. It was. She ran a magnet down my back to release the trapped emotion and that was it. So, so simple.

I walked away thinking, 'That was cool, but now what? What did that do for me?'

I will tell you what it did for me....

I was finishing up a very poor swim season with my three oldest children. I considered it a total waste of money because the children had fought me constantly, whining the whole time.

That summer, I hated swim lessons. I found myself getting anxious every time a lesson was going to start and if there was a reasonable excuse to miss the lessons altogether, we would.

Then Aunt Gwen worked on me. The swim season ended. I didn't think much more about it. But

I started to feel a mysterious and subtle change within myself that I couldn't explain.

The following year, we tried swim lessons again. I was suddenly very much aware of a difference. Without that terrifying memory from my childhood, I wasn't anxious around the water.

In fact, I enjoyed going to the pool. I used the time to catch up on my reading while the children took their lessons.

What amazed me even more, was the change in my children.

Some people may say it was because they were now a year older and so they weren't as frightened of swimming. But I would have to disagree. By clearing a very real emotion that was stuck within me, I know I not only freed myself, but I freed my children as well. - Holly B.

Muscle testing provides a real window into what is going on in the mindbody. Using muscle testing, we can literally gain access to our body's internal computer system and find out where the imbalances are.

I refer to it as *asking the body* what it knows. I've used it for many years in my practice because it leads directly to the root of the problem very quickly. The body-computer always knows, because it is linked into what is often called Universal Consciousness – the database of all that is.

No matter how many times I demonstrate it, people are always impressed by how immediate and accurate muscle testing is. They're amazed by how much their inner mind knows, and how ready it is to give them the information they ask for.

Your Body Knows Best

When it comes to our health, what our bodies can reveal to us is vastly more significant than what we ever know in our conscious minds. During my years in practice, I grew to appreciate the subconscious intelligence of my patients, which nearly always knew what was wrong and what the body needed.

Think about it. Our bodies are tuned into the systems that keep our eyes blinking and our lungs expanding with air. Our subconscious minds are constantly monitoring the white blood cells in our veins and the beating of our hearts. Thankfully, those systems are unconscious to us. But it's only logical that our internal computer would be perfectly aware of exactly what's happening inside of us on every level, all the time.

Not only that, but our bodies can tell us exactly what's good for us and what isn't. We even have a physical response when we tell the truth or a lie. The muscles are instantly weakened when we lie. They stay strong when we tell the truth.

We can't fool our bodies. Our subconscious minds know in an instant, without a doubt, whether we are being true or false — whether we are acting with integrity — in our thoughts, our statements, our actions and our health.

In order to keep us healthy and alive, our bodies use skills that far exceed anything we're consciously aware of. To prove it, psychiatrist Dr. David Hawkins used to offer the 1000 or more people who attended his lectures a vivid demonstration.

Inner Knowing

His staff would pass out sealed, unmarked envelopes to every person in the audience. Each sealed envelope contained a powdery substance. In half of the envelopes, that powder was an artificial sweetener. In the other half, it was organic Vitamin C.

Dr. Hawkins would then ask everyone in the audience to pair up and use a simple muscle testing technique. One person would hold the unmarked envelope over their heart while their partner tested their muscle strength. They would make note of whether the muscle was strong or weak, then they would switch roles and compare. Sometimes the muscles would test weak and sometimes they'd test strong.

Once everyone had completed the simple test, they would open the envelopes to see whether they were holding the artificial sweetener or the Vitamin C.

Every single time the muscles went weak, the person was holding the artificial sweetener. When the muscles tested strong, they were invariably holding an envelope containing Vitamin C. These results were always consistent, and in my own lectures I have found them to be quite repeatable.[1]

We all know that organic Vitamin C is better for us than an artificial sweetener, but the fact that the human body on some deeper level knows what is inside a sealed envelope is truly astounding.

Dr. Hawkins explains it in this way:

The individual human mind is like a computer terminal connected to a giant database. The database is human consciousness itself, of which our own consciousness is merely an individual expression, but with its roots in the common consciousness of all mankind.

This database is the realm of genius; because to be human is to participate in the database, everyone by virtue of his birth has access to genius. The unlimited information contained in the database has now been shown to be readily available to anyone in a few seconds, at any time and in any place. This is indeed an astonishing discovery, bearing the power

---

1 David R. Hawkins, *Power vs. Force: the hidden determinants of human behavior,* (Carlsbad, CA: Hay House, Inc. 1995), 59.

to change lives, both individually and collectively, to a degree never yet anticipated.[2]

Testing Other People

Muscle testing can also be used to find out what is going on in someone else's body. You can do that either by testing the person directly or by using what is known as surrogate or proxy testing. We will talk about those testing methods in chapter 8.

Thousands of vitalistic physicians and practitioners use muscle testing to help their patients on a daily basis.

You can easily learn it and use it to help yourself, your friends and your loved ones to identify and release trapped emotions using the Emotion Code.

Here are a few of the easiest and most common methods of muscle testing someone else:

The Basic Arm Test (to test another person)

First of all, ask the person you wish to test if they have pain in either shoulder. If they do, don't use that arm as it may aggravate their condition. If they have trouble in both shoulders or if they are too young, too weak, or too ill to be tested, you should find a different way to test them using one of the testing methods outlined in this chapter, or you can use a surrogate person to test them (see chapter 8).

2 Ibid, 34.

1 Ask the subject you wish to test to stand up and hold one arm out directly in front of them, horizontal to the floor. They should not make a tight fist, but let their hand remain relaxed.

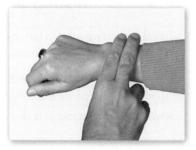

2 Place the first two fingers of one hand lightly on their arm, just above the wrist as shown.

Finger Positioning for Basic Arm Test

3 Place your free hand on their opposite shoulder to support them.

4 Tell the subject "I'm going to have you make a statement, and then I'm going to press down on your arm. I want you to resist me by holding your arm right where it is; try to prevent me from pushing your arm down."

5 Have the subject state their name. If the subject's name is Kim, for example, he or she would say, "My name is Kim."

6 Perform the muscle test by smoothly and steadily increasing the pressure downward on the subjects' arm, going from no pressure to a fairly firm pressure within about 3 seconds.

7 The shoulder joint should stay 'locked' against your firm downward pressure, and should not give way.

A person's arm can rapidly become tired if you overdo the amount of force you use. Remember that muscle testing does not require brute force.

If the statement they just made is true, you should feel that the arm is "locked" against your downward pressure. If the statement is false, you should feel their arm begin to give way under your smoothly increasing pressure.

You should always use the minimum force needed to perceive whether the arm is staying *locked* or not. That is what you are looking for.

Now repeat the test, but have the subject make a statement that is obviously false by using a name that is not their own. Immediately perform the muscle test again, and you should notice the arm is weaker, since the statement just made is incongruent with truth, and the subject's subconscious mind knows it.

Tips on the Basic Arm Test

Here are some tips that will help you to improve and become proficient at muscle testing.

1 Don't use too much force, only what you need to get your answer. Think finesse, not force.

2 Smoothly increase the force from zero to firm over about three seconds.

3 Keep your fingers in the correct position. If you place your fingers on the bones of their wrist, their arm will weaken because the body will attempt to protect the wrist bones. You want your fingers to be just above the wrist bones. Your fingers should be placed just above the bony prominence that can be found on the back of your hand on the little finger side, just above the wrist. (See photo)

4 Remember that the person you are testing has to be willing to be tested. If their attitude is cynical or skeptical, it will be harder for you to test them. Don't waste your time with people that don't want to be helped, or that are not open to being helped. Life is too short.

5 You can experiment with various arm positions to see what works best for you and whomever you are working on. Another option is for them to hold their arm out to the side rather than straight out in front of them.

Testing Yourself

Now let's take a look at some ways of using your own muscles to get answers.

As you try out these methods, it's easiest to make statements that you already know to be true or false. That way you can know with certainty if it is working for you.

In chapter two you learned to do the Sway Test by saying the words "unconditional love" or "hatred." Those words are very powerful and will elicit a definite response from the body.

"Unconditional love" will make you sway forward, and will make any muscle test strong. "Hatred" has just the opposite effect and will weaken you.

The words "yes" and "no" will have similar effects. The word "yes" is positive. If you make a statement that is true or positive, you will test strong, or you will sway forward. "No" is a negative word. If you make a statement that is untrue or negative, you will be weak, or sway backward.

Self-testing methods are more subjective than any of the other methods we have discussed, and are therefore a bit more challenging to learn. I have found that children can learn these methods without any trouble in most cases, but sometimes adults take a bit longer. Some self-testing methods seem to naturally work better for some people than others. Try them out and see what you like. To become proficient at any of these self-testing methods takes time and practice. The main challenge is learning to allow your conscious control to recede a bit into the background, so your body can respond as it will.

Have you ever used a dimmer switch? You might have one on a wall in your home, but if not, you have probably used one before. By turning the knob on a dimmer switch, you can choose exactly how much electricity a light fixture is getting, and therefore how bright it is. With the exception of the Sway Test, the key to all self-testing methods is finding the precise muscle strength setting in your resistance finger.

Hand Solo Method

This method looks a little funny but is actually quite easy to use and can be done with one hand. It happens to be my personal favorite.

You will use two fingers of the same hand. For most people, the forefinger and middle finger work just fine, but if for some reason they don't, then try the middle finger and the ring finger.

Essentially, one finger will assume the role of the arm being tested, (we'll call this the resistance finger) and

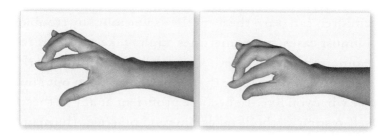

the other finger acts to apply very slight downward pressure to perform the testing (we'll call this the testing finger).

First of all, decide what two fingers feel comfortable when one finger is placed atop the other. Whatever feels best will probably work.

Now place your attention on the finger that is going to be pressed down upon (the resistance finger).

Like turning up a dimmer switch all the way, turn up the muscle tightness in this particular finger all the way, so it is as strong as you can make it.

While maintaining this strength in the resistance finger, press down gently with the testing finger. You will find that nothing happens; the resistance finger will not depress. That's fine.

Now, like turning down a dimmer switch almost all the way, turn down the muscle tone or tightness to the resistance finger, so it is just strong enough to hold its straight-out, straight-line position.

Now, while maintaining this low level of strength in the resistance finger, press down gently with the testing finger. You will find that the resistance finger depresses easily. Again, that's fine.

So far, so good. Here is the important thing to understand.

Self-testing works a little differently than the other types of testing we have learned. The essential difference is that you have to discover your own "dimmer-switch" setting. In other words, you have to learn how strong to make your resistance finger so that congruency will test strong, yet incongruence will test weak. Ready? Here is how to figure it out. It's not hard.

Start by dialing up the muscle strength to your resistance finger to 100%. Nice and strong. Now, simply say the word "no", or you can say, "hatred" and press down with your testing finger. You should notice, with the strength of the resistance finger dialed up all the way, that even when you are saying a negative word, your finger will not depress.

Ah. But now let's try dialing the strength setting on the resistance back a bit. And repeat the negative word, either "no" or "hatred" (either of these words will work, but for the sake of consistency pick one and stay with it while you are learning this). Now press down on the resistance finger, and see what happens. Nothing? No problem.

Try setting the muscle tone on the resistance finger back a bit more, and repeat the negative word, then test again.

And so on. At some point, you will find a dimmer-switch/muscle strength setting for your resistance finger that is just weak enough that it will give way under the pressure of the testing finger when you say one of these negative words. As soon as this happens, use that strength setting in the resistance finger and say something positive, such as "yes" or "love", and immediately test again. It should test strong.

The whole key to this method of self-testing is to figure out how strong you need to make your resistance finger so that it will stay strong on a positive word like love, and go weak on a negative word like hatred. That is all there is to it, really.

Some people can pick up self-testing very easily. The most difficult thing about this type of testing is its subjective nature.

The human tendency is to question every answer you get when you are testing yourself, but you need to simply trust yourself and trust your subconscious mind, where the answers are coming from.

I have found self-testing to be invaluable. It takes practice, and may seem impossible at first, but if you will stay with it, I think you will find it to be invaluable as well.

Falling Log Method

If you were to use the Hand Solo method of self-testing, but with two hands instead of one, it would look like this next method.

If you are right-handed, make a fist with your left hand, and extend your left forefinger straight out. This finger will be your resistance finger, or the finger that will be tested.

Place your right hand over your fist and grip it firmly, placing the last joint of your right pinky finger atop your out-stretched left forefinger in whatever position feels comfortable. If you are left-handed, just reverse your hand positions.

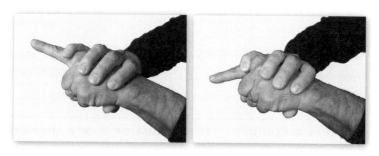

Now that you have your fingers positioned correctly, you can follow the same pattern that I gave you in the Hand Solo explanation. For your convenience, I will give you those same instructions right here:

Start by dialing up the muscle strength to your resistance finger to 100%. Nice and strong. Now, simply say the word "no", or you can say, "hatred" and press down with your testing finger. You should notice, with the strength of the resistance finger dialed up all the way, that even when you are saying a negative word, your finger will not depress.

Now let's try dialing the strength setting on the resistance back a bit. Now repeat the negative word, either "no" or "hatred." Try setting the muscle tone on the resistance finger back a bit more, and repeat the negative word, then test again.

At some point as you continue this process, you will find a dimmer-switch/muscle strength setting for your resistance finger that is just weak enough, and it will give way under the pressure of the testing finger when you say one of these negative words. As soon as this happens, use that strength setting in the resistance finger and say something positive, such as "yes" or "love", and immediately test again. It should test strong.

Hole-In-One Method

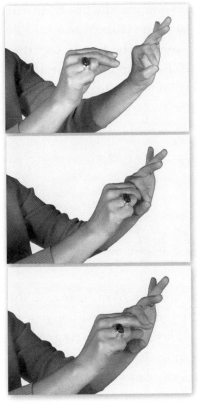

With one hand, make an OK sign, by touching the tip of your thumb to the tip of your forefinger. Then slide the thumb and the first two fingers of your opposite hand into that ring. The fingers inside the ring will be the testing fingers. The fingers that are forming the ring will be the resistance fingers.

Following the procedure I have outlined in the previous two methods, try varying the amount of resistance in the ring, while saying something negative or incongruent. As you make the statement, use the fingers inside the ring to press outward. Try to press hard enough to pull the ring apart. Resist that pressure with the fingers making the ring. When you find the strength setting that gives you weakness on a negative or incongruent statement, and yet remains strong on a positive or congruent statement, you are there.

Linked Rings Method

Make a ring with the thumb and middle finger on one hand. Now, make a ring with the thumb and middle finger of the other hand, joining the hands together like two links in a chain. The thumb and forefinger that are forming one of the rings will be the resistance fingers.

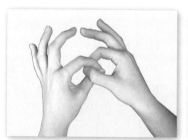 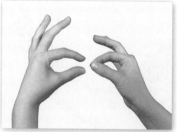

Once again, try varying the amount of resistance in the rings, while saying something negative or incongruent. As you make the statement, try to pull the rings apart. Remember that you are simply attempting to find the strength setting that allows the rings to pull apart on a negative or incongruent statement, and remain linked on a positive or congruent statement.

Finding One That Works for You

I have found that around 80% of the people in my live seminars will have immediate success using at least one of the self-testing methods I have described in this chapter. My advice to you is to simply practice.

Don't give up! While some people seem to pick up these self-testing methods instantly, most people have to practice. Just stick with it for a while, and like riding a bike, it will become second nature to you before long.

If one of these testing methods is more comfortable or feels more natural to you, practice it.

By only using words that are clearly positive or negative such as yes/no or love/hate while you are learning, you'll be able to refine this skill much more quickly. Learning self-testing is optional to using the Emotion Code, but mastery of any self-testing method can make things easier and more efficient for you.

Of course, the simplest self-testing method is the Sway Test, which takes very little practice for most people. The only drawbacks to the Sway Test are that you must be standing to use it, and that it takes a bit more time than the other self-testing methods, as you need to allow the body time to sway without forcing it.

When I became proficient at self-testing I saw the advantages immediately. I no longer needed another person to help me test patients who were temporarily untestable. I could test them on myself now. I could also check myself for trapped emotions and other imbalances and correct them myself. Self-testing gave me a very rapid, effective and simple way to get to the answers I was looking for.

If It Hurts, Stop!

If any of these tests begin to cause even the slightest discomfort, switch to a different test. Discomfort or pain is a sign that you are using too much force, and if you continue in spite of the discomfort, you could injure yourself or create inflammation in the tissues.

Ideally you should use the least amount of muscle strength necessary to perform any form of muscle testing. When I was learning these methods for the first time, I used too high a strength setting, and the result was sore fingers. I eventually found that I could use a muscle strength setting that was barely enough to hold up my resistance finger. These self-testing methods will work at different resistance strengths, but the higher the resistance, the more tiring the testing will be for you, and the more likely your fingers will become sore. If you experience discomfort in performing any of these tests, stop. Choose a different method of testing until the soreness goes away, and try using less resistance.

Training Wheels and Intuition

If you use the Emotion Code for very long, you may begin to notice an odd phenomenon. A split-second before you get an answer through muscle testing, the answer may suddenly appear in your mind, like a quiet little voice whispering to you. At first, it might be so quiet that you might overlook it.

You may not be used to listening to this little voice, but you may find yourself saying, "I knew that was the answer." Just as you are beginning to do the test, you'll just feel it and know. This intuitive knowledge flows into you from the universal database of consciousness, from the sea of intelligence and energy that surrounds us all.

Muscle testing is like training-wheels for your intuition.

As you become more adept at listening to your intuition, you will find that you *can* know what the answer is in this way. You can feel it. The more heed you give to these subtle promptings, the better you will get at knowing the answers to your questions.

Nonverbal Communication

The communication that takes place between you as the healer and your subject does not necessarily have to be verbal. I stumbled across this phenomenon myself many years ago. I was used to using leg-length testing as my primary method of evaluating patients, and I had used it successfully for many years. Leg-length testing takes a bit more time to learn and master, so I will not be teaching it here, but it can be learned by going to _HealersLibrary.com_.

Leg-length testing is really just another form of muscle testing, but the answers are given by the body through changes in the leg-length instead of changes in muscle strength. I quickly learned that the body would give me answers just as easily using this form of testing as with any other form. It became my primary method of getting answers from my patient's bodies. In fact, for many years the very first thing that I did with most patients was to have them lie face down and simply ask their body for a "yes" or a "no" answer, which the body would give through changes in the leg-length. The legs would be even in length for "yes" and uneven for "no." It always worked for me, without any trouble, but one day something interesting happened.

I had been working on a patient for a few minutes, and his treatment was drawing to a close. I looked down and checked his leg-length, and it was perfectly balanced. I looked up at his back, and idly turned my attention to his _right_ kidney. I thought about his right kidney for a moment. Then I looked down and checked his leg length again. Suddenly his leg-length was dramatically different. I relaxed my grip, looked up and thought about his _left_ kidney this time. I rechecked his leg-length, and his legs were balanced.

I again thought about his *right* kidney for a moment, rechecked, and the leg-length difference was obvious. I was amazed! As you might imagine, this patient did have something going on in his right kidney. In fact, it turned out that he had a trapped emotion embedded in that area of his body, imbalancing his right kidney. Immediately after releasing this trapped emotion, I could no longer get his leg length to change by merely contemplating his right kidney, since the reason for the kidney imbalance was gone.

This experience was a bit of an epiphany for me, and I immediately put this knowledge to use. From that point on, it became standard procedure for me to ask questions of the body silently. The results were the same as before. The only difference was that I was now merely thinking the questions that before I had been thinking *and* vocalizing.

I never had any problem with this kind of testing for many years. It seemed to me that there was a full and complete communication link between my patients and myself that was entirely nonverbal.

I found that any question I could ask out loud could be asked silently with no difference in the result.

By the way, nonverbal communication works with all forms of testing, from the Sway Test to the Basic Arm Test, to every other method I have ever seen.

The person being tested can simply think their statement, and the result will be the same as if they had vocalized the question. By the same token, the person doing the testing can simply think the question they want to ask the subject, and the result will be as if they had vocalized the question.

I never had any problem with this kind of nonverbal testing until one particular patient helped me to learn an important lesson.

The Clown from Hell

Bill had come to me for treatment of his low back pain a few months before. He was doing very well, and on this particular day he had come in for a routine check up. He lay face down on my adjusting table and I performed a leg-length test on him. I directed my thoughts toward his body and thought, "Give me a Yes answer." I checked his leg length. It was balanced. Then I thought, "Give me a No answer." I checked his leg length again, but to my surprise, there was no change. This was very odd. I had been using this type of testing for over a decade, but I had never seen this happen. His leg length should have changed, but it didn't. I couldn't understand why it wasn't working.

I repeated the procedure several times with no change. Puzzled, I looked up from his feet for a moment and noticed what was on his back. He was wearing a white T-shirt, and on the back was a shockingly evil image of a clown face, with fangs dripping blood.

On a hunch, I got a piece of paper and covered the image with it. Then I retested his leg length, and suddenly the testing worked as it should. I was frankly amazed. I uncovered the image, tried the testing again, and… nothing. I covered the image with the paper again, and he was testable. So far, not a word had passed between the two of us since I had begun testing.

After removing and replacing the paper a few more times, each time confirming the result, I finally told him what was going on. I said, "I think that the clown picture on the back of your t-shirt is affecting you negatively and that you might want to think about getting rid of it." He never returned to my office after that.

Everything that exists radiates vibrational energy that has an ultimate effect on our own energy field, whether good or bad.

Some things will have a more positive vibrational effect, and others will have a more negative one. For example, if you look at a picture of Adolf Hitler, you will probably test weak or sway backward, away from his image and all the negativity that it connotes. If you look at a picture of Mother Teresa, you will very likely test strong, or sway toward her picture, toward all of the positivity of her energy. If you gaze upon a painting of a beautiful countryside, the positive vibrational energy radiated by the painting will have a positive effect on you. On the other hand, a painting of a scene of degradation and evil will vibrate at a much lower frequency, and your body will find it repulsive. I believe that it is the objects themselves that radiate these frequencies, positive or negative. Our personal values and mental associations play a part as well.

Here's a test that you can take that will show you how negativity and positivity affect your energy. Take a look at this simple figure.

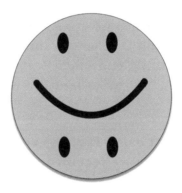

If you hold it one way, it's a positive, smiling face. If you turn it upside down, it becomes a negative, frowning face. If you fix your gaze upon the picture when it is right side up, you will find that you will sway toward it or test strong. If you turn it upside down, you will sway away from it or test weak. Don't take my word for it. Give it a try and see for yourself.

Troubleshooting

Your Subject Suddenly Tests Consistently Weak

The mind does an amazing job keeping track of things, and usually you will be able to clear trapped emotions without the mind needing to take a break. But once in a while, the brain becomes overwhelmed with the myriad bits of interconnected data and the connections and reconnections that need to be made after a trapped emotion is released.

This result is a phenomenon I call "overload", which will make a person test weak no matter what you do. It is a temporary condition, and usually lasts less than 30 seconds.

On rare occasions, (with more severe trapped emotions, typically) I have seen patients go into overload and stay in this state for hours to an entire day. More often, if you just give your subject a minute or so, their brain will finish processing, and they will become testable again.

By way of explanation, imagine the following scenario. You find yourself sitting in your car in the middle of the night. The headlights are on. The engine is off. The car won't start. You turn the key to start the car, and the engine turns over and over, RRRRrrrrr RRRRrrrr RRRRrrrr. You notice that as the engine turns over, the headlights dim. This is similar to what is occurring in the body during overload. As the mind is furiously turning over, processing what you have just done, the amount of energy available for muscle testing is diminished.

Your Subject Tests Strong No Matter What

If you are trying to work with a person that tests strong no matter what you do, consider that this person may be untestable at present. In my experience, about one in fifty people are considered to be temporarily untestable; that is, they will stay strong no matter how incongruent or untrue their statement. It is not a serious problem, however, nor is it permanent.

I've found that this is usually due to one of two things. Either they are dehydrated or one or more bones in their neck is out of alignment.

When someone is dehydrated, it directly affects their muscle strength and their electrical conductivity. Have them drink a glass of water, then try again. Sometimes, that's all it takes. You may also drink some water; if you are dehydrated the testing will be affected in the same way.

If they need a neck adjustment, misaligned bones may be creating interference in the nervous system, inhibiting the nerve connections and throwing off the messages to their muscles. In that case, they should see their chiropractor for an adjustment, after which they should be testable.

Please note that it is always possible to test an untestable person by testing on yourself if you are practiced at it. You can also work around this problem by using surrogate testing, which we'll discuss in more detail in chapter 8. Instead of testing the subject directly, surrogate testing allows you to test a third person and still tap into the subconscious of the subject to get the desired answers.

If someone is determined not to be muscle tested, they will usually succeed.

But that means they're deliberately being uncooperative and don't want the testing to work. They've got their own agenda. If that's the case they're not an ideal candidate for the Emotion Code. Now and then, I've run into people who have already made up their minds that muscle testing doesn't work. And wouldn't you know it? It doesn't work on them! They make sure of that.

As you've seen, these tests are not about sheer physical force. I have seen cases where a person's muscle went so weak that they literally could not resist the slightest downward pressure, but that's not usually the case. More often, what you will detect is a slight change in muscle strength, the difference between the muscle being 'locked' or 'mushy'.

Muscle testing works on most of the people, most of the time. But other things can come into play. Sometimes it doesn't work because they're just not comfortable for some reason. Or they think it's hokey. Or they're defensive, afraid that something might be revealed about them. For example, I have found that sometimes people will be untestable in front of a group of people, yet become perfectly testable when they are no longer in front of an audience.

Always Get Permission

Always explain what you are going to do before you do it. If you are going to be pressing down on their arm to test them, explain the procedure beforehand and get their permission.

It is possible to test other people through self-testing without their knowing it, and this is wrong.

It is critical to ask permission of the person you are going to test, and it is critical that you honor their wishes.

Testing people without their permission or against their wishes is a true invasion of their privacy and is just plain wrong. It's unethical. Don't do it!

Never test or work on a minor without the permission of their parent or guardian!

Muscle Testing is Not for Winning the Lotto

Muscle testing is a gift from God, to allow us to help each other. It is not to be used to test for the winning lotto numbers, it is not to be used to ask if you should take that job, etc. Asking about anything unrelated to health probably won't work anyway, in my experience. You can ask about the present, but do not try to see the future, as muscle testing is not for that purpose and the results would be unreliable at best. This kind of testing is for the present, and applies to what is happening now, in the present, as well as determining trapped emotions from the past.

Do Not Use Testing to Make Big Decisions

You will have to trust me on this one. Speaking from experience, it has become clear to me that testing is a gift from God that has a specific purpose, but that purpose is limited. You can muscle test every decision you make, but you won't get anything but neurotic, in my opinion. Use muscle testing to find trapped emotions and to help yourself and others to get and stay physically well and leave it at that.

Allow Yourself to be Guided

Don't be too proud to ask God for help. He already knows the answers you are looking for, and he wants to help you, but you have to ask. I am reminded of the famous painting of Christ, where he is standing at the front door of a home, knocking. The funny thing is, the front door has no doorknob on the outside. He won't open the door. You have to do it. And believe me when I tell you that I utter a silent prayer every single time I test anyone, and I ask God to help me, every single time, and He always does. Try it!

Be Patient With Yourself

Some people grasp these skills very easily while others take more time. I promise you that if you will persevere, it will become easy for you, and it will open a whole world of healing to you.

The first time someone looks into your eyes and thanks you with tears in their eyes for what you have done for them, you will understand what I mean.

There is nothing more addicting than that feeling of helping people. It's the greatest! And it doesn't happen every time, but it will happen if you just have it in your heart to help as many people as you can.

Establish a Baseline

Because people are so different, it's crucial to establish a baseline with every person so that you know what congruency or incongruence feels like in their particular case.

The simplest way to do this is to have them make a known true statement, then a known false statement, such as stating their name as their own name, then stating their name as the name of someone else, or have them say a positive word such as "yes" or "love", followed by a negative word such as "no" or "hate".

Check Your Work

If during testing I get a strong muscle or a weak muscle three or more times in a row, I like to re-do the baseline test to make sure the person is still testable.

If your testing is taking more time than usual, it's a good idea to check your baseline periodically to make sure you are on track. Sometimes people can go into overload while you're testing them, and in that case, you would get weakness on every test you perform until they are done processing. It's good practice to test them on a negative word if you keep getting strong responses, and vice versa.

Watch Out for Wandering Thoughts

It is possible to influence the outcome of testing by what you are thinking. If you don't believe me, just see what happens when you muscle test someone while thinking something negative or derogatory about them. They will be weak. It is really important to stay focused.

If you are holding negative thoughts in your head about the person you're testing — even if that person is you — the muscles can easily pick that up and go weak.

Positive intentions and clarity are very important to getting accurate tests. Keep it simple, focus on the statement that has just been made, and keep other thoughts out of your mind. Instruct the person you are testing to do the same.

Allow love to fill your heart for the person you are trying to help. Have a sincere desire to help them. Believe that you can do it and be grateful to God that you are *doing* it. That's all it takes.

Don't Diagnose Unless You Are a Doctor

If you are a doctor, diagnosing people is what you do. But if you are not a doctor, never diagnose anyone, as that is known as practicing medicine without a license, and is illegal. Be aware of what people are telling you, and if they are having symptoms that seem at all unusual to you, recommend to them that they seek adequate medical attention.

Don't Worry About Non-believers

Not everyone is open to learning about new methods of healing such as the Emotion Code. You may have family members who think you are off your nut, or your dog may leave you. Don't let these things bother you. The greatest healer in history was Jesus, and very few believed him, so you are in good company.

Who or What Are We Asking When We Test?

We're talking to the subconscious mind. The way I look at it, there is no difference between this and the spirit or higher intelligence in all of us. Somehow this part of us is linked to the intelligence of God and the

Universe, and somehow muscle testing seems to tap into these as well.

The Veil of Memory

When you work on someone, you are really working on a dual-natured being that has a physical body and a spirit. I believe that when we come into this world there's a veil placed over our minds, so we have no memory of our previous existence. We arrive with complete amnesia.

Allow me to share with you a very personal experience about this concept.

One day as I sat quietly in meditation I had a profound spiritual insight.

The veil of memory that divides us from our existence before we came here to this earth was suddenly broken for me. Every particle of my being was instantaneously filled with an overwhelming and indescribably powerful feeling of *homesickness*. Homesickness to be *back* in my heavenly home, my *real home* where I came from. This impossibly intense feeling only lasted for a few seconds, and then was gone, leaving me reeling with awe.

I've experienced over the years of my life that feeling that we call homesickness on a number of occasions, but the homesickness I experienced in this spiritual revelation was far beyond anything that I can even describe to you.

I realized from this experience that this veil of forgetfulness is a good thing. If we didn't have it to block us from the memories of our glorious past when we lived with our Heavenly Father, I'm convinced we would not be able to endure this earth life for five minutes.

I realized from this experience that we truly are strangers here; that "trailing clouds of glory do we come from God, who is our home."

The earth is not really our home; we are sojourners here, sent here to choose between good and evil; sent here to gain faith and to gain the experience of living in physical bodies. We are sent here to learn to love and serve one another. By doing so, we serve God.

At some level, your spirit is in touch with things that are beyond the comprehension of your conscious mind. But your spirit can speak to you through your physical body. Muscle testing is the conduit that enables you to tap into that knowledge.

I believe that we have always existed, and that more profound knowledge lies deep within our minds than we can consciously know.

Isn't it great that all we have to do is ask?

FAITH IS TO BELIEVE WHAT WE DO NOT SEE;
AND THE REWARD OF THIS FAITH
IS TO SEE WHAT WE BELIEVE.

- SAINT AUGUSTINE

6

RELEASING TRAPPED EMOTIONS

Now that you've had an opportunity to learn about and practice muscle testing, it's time to learn the part of the Emotion Code that deals with finding and releasing trapped emotions, both from yourself and from others.

You will find that this process is simple and logical. Once you have been through it a few times, you will become more efficient. With practice, most people can find and release a trapped emotion in less than a minute or two.

First of all, make sure that you (and your partner, if applicable) are comfortable in your environment. It's best to turn off music and television, as they can be distracting and can have negative or positive energetic effects of their own.

The Emotion Code process can be visualized using the graphic image below.

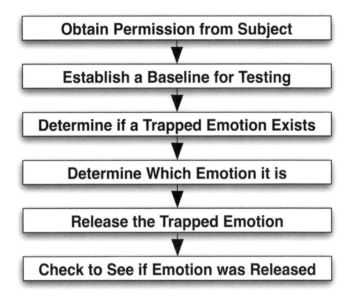

Obtain Permission from Subject

Establish a Baseline for Testing

Determine if a Trapped Emotion Exists

Determine Which Emotion it is

Release the Trapped Emotion

Check to See if Emotion was Released

Step 1: Obtain Permission

If you're working on yourself, you already have permission, so go to the next step.

If you are going to be working with another person, make sure that you get permission to actually test them and get information from their body. You might ask, "Can I have your permission to test you for trapped emotions?" Don't muscle test this response. Let your partner give you their verbal okay, or at least nod their assent.

Once you both feel comfortable and are relaxed, you can begin.

Step 2: Establish a Baseline

Before you begin to ask about trapped emotions, your first task is to establish a baseline for testing. Choose the muscle testing method that you are most comfortable using. You need to determine if your subject is testable. If they make a congruent or true statement, are they strong? If they make an incongruent or false statement, are they weak?

In addition, since every person is unique, muscle testing will feel slightly different for each person you test. Getting a definite strong and weak muscle response from your partner will immediately let you know just what this particular person's muscle test feels like in both strong and weak states.

Perhaps the most obvious and widely used method of establishing a baseline is to simply have your partner state their own name by saying out loud, "My name is _____."

Once they have made this congruent or true statement, they should test strong.

Now have your partner make a false statement by saying out loud, "My name is _____", filling in the blank with any name that is not their own. The result should be muscle weakness.

Of course, having your partner state the words yes or no, love or hate, will also work for establishing a baseline.

If Your Partner is Untestable

Remember that part of the reason for establishing a baseline is to determine if the person you are working with is currently *testable*. If their arm stays strong or weak, no matter what statement they make, they are untestable at present. In this case, you have certain options.

If either you or your partner is somewhat dehydrated it will make testing more difficult, if not impossible.

Mild dehydration is quite common and is easily remedied. Give them a glass of water, drink a glass yourself and try again. If this doesn't help, your partner likely has a misaligned vertebra in their neck. You can use a surrogate to test them, or you can test them on yourself until they can get an adjustment from their chiropractor.

Some people are untestable because they have a physical impairment or limitation, and surrogate testing is the best option for helping them as well. For more detailed information on surrogate testing, see chapter 8.

Step 3: See if a Trapped Emotion Exists

Have the person being tested make this statement: "I have a trapped emotion that can be released now."

Test for the response by whatever method you have chosen. Here is a table of the possible methods and possible results.

Test	Yes	No
All Muscle Tests	Strength	Weakness
Sway Test	Forward	Back

If the body's answer is No, there are three distinct possibilities.

1 The first possibility is that the subject doesn't have any trapped emotions at all. This is very unlikely, since nearly everyone has them.

2 The second possibility may be that the subject *has* a trapped emotion, but for some reason their subconscious mind does not want to *release* it right now. This was the statement: "I have a trapped emotion that can be released *now*." The subject may be willing, but their subconscious mind may not be. This situation can change, and the answer may be different later on.

3 The third possibility is that the subject has a *Heart-Wall*. If this is the case, the body may say that it doesn't have any trapped emotions, when in reality it does. The Heart-Wall has the effect of making all trapped emotions a little harder to find. To avoid confusion, I am going to devote the entire next chapter to the Heart-Wall. My recommendation is to go ahead and read through this chapter

now, even if the answer you got is no, as you will need to know the procedure anyway.

If the answer is yes, you can proceed to the next step.

Step 4: Determine Which Emotion It Is

If the answer is yes, there is a trapped emotion to be released. The next step is to learn more about this emotion. What emotion is this? Is it anger? Is it sorrow? Is it frustration or depression, or some other emotion? When did this emotion become trapped? What event created this?

Through a simple process of deduction, you can narrow it down very quickly.

The "Chart of Emotions" shown on the next page is designed to make your task even easier.

Let's take a look at this chart. Notice that each row contains specific emotions produced by one of two organs. For example, Row 1 lists the emotions produced by the Heart or Small Intestine. As you may recall, all emotions emanate from the organs, and these two organs produce the same emotions in the body. All the other organs listed on the chart produce the emotions in their respective rows. For our purposes, it doesn't matter which organ a trapped emotion originally emanated from, as long as we can identify the emotion and release it.

After you've been through this process a few times, it will become quite rapid and simple. You will be amazed to see how quickly you can discover for yourself exactly

The Emotion Code™ Chart		
	Column A	Column B
Row 1 Heart or Small Intestine	Abandonment Betrayal Forlorn Lost Love Unreceived	Effort Unreceived Heartache Insecurity Overjoy Vulnerability
Row 2 Spleen or Stomach	Anxiety Despair Disgust Nervousness Worry	Failure Helplessness Hopelessness Lack of Control Low Self-Esteem
Row 3 Lung or Colon	Crying Discouragement Rejection Sadness Sorrow	Confusion Defensiveness Grief Self-Abuse Stubborness
Row 4 Liver or Gall Bladder	Anger Bitterness Guilt Hatred Resentment	Depression Frustration Indecisiveness Panic Taken for Granted
Row 5 Kidneys or Bladder	Blaming Dread Fear Horror Peeved	Conflict Creative Insecurity Terror Unsupported Wishy Washy
Row 6 Glands & Sexual Organs	Humiliation Jealousy Longing Lust Overwhelm	Pride Shame Shock Unworthy Worthless

which trapped emotion you are seeking. Remember that the subconscious mind knows all along what the trapped emotion is. The testing you are doing is simply to determine what the subconscious mind already knows.

In fact, the subconscious mind of the person you are working on can somehow "see" the chart of emotions without their ever having seen it physically! It's best, in fact, if the person you are working on cannot see the emotion list while you are working on them. Otherwise, they may "choose" an emotion to go weak or strong on, thinking they are helping you out, when they are just skewing the testing. If you want to show them the chart of emotions once at the beginning of a session, that's okay. And even if they have *never* seen the chart themselves, their subconscious mind will "read" the chart just fine, because their subconscious mind is linked into universal consciousness. Try it and see.

Finding the Correct Column

Begin the process of questioning by asking, "Is this trapped emotion listed in Column A?" and then perform the test. If the answer is "Yes", you might want to ask, "Is this trapped emotion in Column B?" to get a "No" answer and check your accuracy.

You will always only be searching for one trapped emotion at a time, and it can only be in one of the two columns. As a result, only one of these questions can possibly be true.

If the body gives a conflicting response such as telling you that the trapped emotion is in both column A and column B, you are just not getting a good answer. Take a deep breath, get refocused, fill your heart with love for the person you are trying to help, (yourself, if you are working on yourself) say a silent prayer to God for help, believe you can get an accurate response, be grateful that the answer is there to find, and try again. Note that if the exact emotion is not listed on this chart, the subconscious mind of the person you are working on will choose the emotion that is closest to the one that is trapped, and as a result this chart should be all you will need.

Finding the Correct Row

Once you have determined which column the trapped emotion is in, you have narrowed the list by half. Now let's determine which row it's in.

We could simply start at the top and ask one row at a time, but to speed it up, I have numbered the rows one through six. So, instead of asking about each row, we can eliminate some rows right away.

Ask, "Is the trapped emotion in an odd-numbered row?" If the answer is no, then you know that it must be in row two, four or six. If the answer is yes, you know it is in an odd-numbered row. For the purpose of our explanation here, we will assume that the emotion is in an odd numbered row, either one, three or five. The next thing we must determine is which row the trapped emotion is listed in.

Ask this question: "Is this trapped emotion listed in row one?" If the answer is no, ask the same question about row three, and row five if you need to.

Finding the Correct Emotion

Once you have identified the correct row, since you already have identified the column, you now have narrowed the list of emotions to five possibilities.

Let's say for example you have determined that the trapped emotion is in column A row 5. Let's take a look at that particular cell in the table.

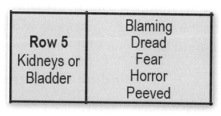

Again, the *subconscious* mind of the person you are testing knows precisely which one of these trapped emotions you are after.

By determining through muscle testing exactly which emotion it is, you bring the knowledge of this trapped emotion to the awareness of your subject's conscious mind.

This is a necessary and indispensable step towards releasing the emotion. It's important for the trapped emotion to find *expression* in order to be released. By identifying it and bringing it to consciousness, we are validating the emotion and bringing a degree of closure to the situation that created it.

We are giving the trapped emotion a voice, and allowing it to be heard, in a sense. If we *don't* do this, the trapped emotion will continue to make its presence felt by creating physical pain and/or emotional dysfunction.

In order to find out exactly which emotion has become trapped, all you need to do is ask.

For example, in this case you could begin by asking "Is this trapped emotion blaming?" and then perform a muscle test. The answer will be either yes or no.

Test each emotion one at a time in this same way until you feel confident that you have arrived at the correct emotion. If the very first emotion on the list is giving you a yes answer, you would be wise to check your work by testing the next emotion on the list, which should give you a no answer. Remember, you are testing for one emotion at a time, no more, and only one should be positive at a time.

It is important to be clear about what you are asking. Your intention and the words that you are saying need to be in synch. This is something to be aware of, so that you don't confuse the subconscious mind.

In addition, cast away any anxiety you may have about this process. Anxiety is a form of fear, and faith and fear cannot coexist!

How to Ask

It's best to frame things in the form of a statement or a question. To illustrate what I mean, imagine that the trapped emotion is *dread*. In this case, you could say "This trapped emotion is dread." and you would get a yes answer.

If you put it in the form of a question and ask, "Is this trapped emotion dread?" you would also get a yes answer.

Both of these ways of asking are equivalent, and each form of phrasing will give you the same body response.

If you just went down the list and stated the word "dread," without formatting it as either a statement or a question, you may get a confused answer. The body may sway backward or test weak when you just say, "dread", even in a situation where dread is the precise emotion that is trapped. If you just throw the word out there, the subconscious mind may not be reading you correctly and may simply respond to the negative energy of the word itself.

Once the Trapped Emotion is Identified

Once you have identified the trapped emotion, congratulations! You have learned a very significant part of the Emotion Code. You have now been introduced to an entirely different aspect of your awareness, and you are now learning to tap into your own spirit intelligence, an ability that will serve you well if you continue to develop it.

Digging Deeper

Sometimes the subconscious mind has more information it wants to push up to the conscious level before being willing to release the emotion. At this point it is a good idea to ask, "Is there more that we need to know about this trapped emotion?" If the answer is no, go ahead and release the emotion. If the answer is yes, dig a little deeper.

Engaging the conscious mind in the process is useful, and can help the subject to grasp the relevance of the emotion that's about to be released.

Remember that the subconscious mind knows all there is to know about this trapped emotion, including when it first became trapped in the body, who was involved, exactly where this energy is lodged and how it is affecting both the physical body and the mind.

If the subconscious mind wants to have more about the trapped emotion brought to conscious awareness, I recommend that you first try to find out when the it originally became trapped. Sometimes this leads to surprising revelations about the past, and will often uncover the event that created the trapped emotion.

When Did it Become Trapped?

Asking *when* this particular emotion became trapped is a good place to begin digging deeper. There are many ways of asking deductive questions to get to this information, and if you have a hunch, follow it.

For example, if finding a trapped emotion brings to mind a certain event from the subject's life, it probably became trapped because of that event. To find out, simply ask if the event that your partner has in mind is the same event that helped to create the trapped emotion. Your partner does not need to share anything about the experience with you if they don't wish to. They just need to think about the event for a moment, and then you need to muscle test them after asking if that event helped to create the trapped emotion.

This is one of the nice things about the Emotion Code. People's private matters can remain private.

They never have to explain or vocalize the circumstance or event that created the trapped emotion. This allows people to work on very private issues that are potentially painful or embarrassing to talk about and still release the emotions that are attached to these events. They can share us much or as little as they choose to.

If no particular event comes to your partner's mind regarding the emotion, you can use the process of deduction to determine when the trapped emotion occurred. Finding out *when* it occurred often helps in uncovering *why* it occurred.

In the same way that we divided the Chart of Emotions into columns and rows to facilitate faster searching, you can divide a lifetime into different spans to more easily locate the year a trapped emotion originated.

There is no right or wrong way to determine when an emotion became trapped. You simply ask, and narrow it down to a certain year or event. One way to do it is to simply divide your subject's span of years in two, and see if the trapped emotion occurred before the midpoint of their life, or after. If they are forty years old, for example, you might ask, "Did this emotion become trapped before age twenty?" If the answer is yes, you can narrow it down further in this same way.

You might ask, "Did this emotion become trapped within the first ten years of your (my) life?"

If the answer is yes, you can break it down even further, by asking:

"Did this emotion become trapped in the first five years of your (my) life?"

If the answer is yes, you can continue to refine the answer by asking if the emotion became trapped in the first year, second year, third year and so on.

I have found that the body is usually accurate within a year plus or minus when identifying the time frame of a trapped emotion in this way. In other words, if you get the answer that a certain trapped emotion occurred at age 17, it could actually have been at age 16 or age 18, but it probably was at age 17.

At the moment a trapped emotion is being created your particular age is apparently not all that important. The mindbody doesn't correlate trapped emotions with chronological age so much as it correlates them with specific events, occurrences or circumstances.

Let's say an emotional event that occurred a month after you graduated from college resulted in a trapped emotion. You happened to be 23 years old at the time. Muscle testing may produce an answer of 22, 23 or 24 years old for when this trapped emotion occurred, which would be within the usual year, plus or minus. If you were to ask if this trapped emotion occurred before graduation, or after graduation, you would get a more precise answer. In this way, you would be able to arrive at a more accurate time of occurrence.

It's good practice to periodically ask, "Do we need to know more about this emotion?" When you've brought enough information about the trapped emotion to consciousness, the mindbody will let you know you're done, and it can be released.

Once you've determined exactly when the emotion occurred, your subject will probably know what event helped create it and what it was about.

Sometimes, determining the time frame when a trapped emotion occurred can result in a more profound understanding of what happened, as well as how the trapped emotion is affecting the mindbody. Here is an account of a woman who developed a trapped emotion during a stressful time, which led to migraine headaches later on.

Nancy's Migraines

I was always getting very bad headaches and bad neck aches, and I had even started getting cortisone shots in the back of my head and neck. When you said that I might have a trapped emotion that was causing this, I had no clue what you were talking about. You started asking my body questions like something happened to me in 1994. You narrowed it down to an emotion of hopelessness in the month of January, 1994.

Then I started thinking, 'Oh my gosh, this is the time Shawn was born when I went into labor at 33 weeks.' He was in the Hospital for 21 days with a collapsed lung. After you treated me I feel so much better, and I thank you for that.

What a miracle. I said that you knew I had all this block in the back of my head because we almost lost Shawn during this time. But if you see him, you will know he is truly my miracle.

- Nancy P.

Whose Emotion Was This?

Sometimes it can help to understand who was involved in the creation of a trapped emotion. For example, let's say you are hot on the trail of a trapped emotion that occurred during your high school years. The emotion is bitterness. But you can't remember anything that might have created this emotion.

You might ask, "Was this *my* bitterness?" If the answer is yes, you can ask if the bitterness was toward a person. If it was, you might ask if it was a male? Was it a female? Was it a friend? Was it a family member? Was it your brother? Was it Joe? Use the process of deduction to narrow down the possibilities.

If it was your own bitterness but it was not about a person, you can ask if the bitterness was about a situation. Then narrow your scope of questions to figure out what the situation was, when it occurred, etc.

Emotions rarely occur in a vacuum. They usually involve another person, but can be about a situation regarding home, school, work, finances, relationships, etc.

If you test to see if it was *your* bitterness and the answer is no, then ask if it was someone else's bitterness that you *absorbed* from them. We do take on other people's feelings sometimes, and that energy can become our extra baggage. A mother can be feeling bitterness and her child might pick up some of that energy, or a friend might be going through a difficult episode, and your empathy for her situation may create a trapped emotion for you. In my experience, if an emotion was absorbed from another person, the subconscious mind will always want that fact to be brought to consciousness before the trapped emotion is released.

If you silence your mind for a moment or two, and especially if you ask God for His help to figure it out, you will. Trust me on this. Remember, "Ask, and ye shall receive; knock, and it shall be opened unto you."

Where is the Emotion Lodged?

Another fascinating thing to determine is exactly where the trapped emotion is lodged. Remember that a trapped emotion will always have a physical location in the body. Figuring out where a trapped emotion is located is optional, but locating it can be fun as well as very enlightening.

Trapped emotions can lodge anywhere in the body, regardless of what organ they originated from.

Remember that a trapped emotion is a ball of energy, usually ranging in size from an orange to a cantaloupe. To determine the exact location of this energy ball, use the process of deduction.

Ask, "Is this trapped emotion stuck in the right side of the body?" If not, ask, "Is this trapped emotion stuck in the left side of the body?" Each time you ask, perform the muscle test of your choice to see what the body's answer is.

If both of these answers are negative, ask, "Is this trapped emotion stuck in the midline of the body?"

Next, ask if the trapped emotion is above, below or at the waistline. Before long you will have identified a general area where the emotional energy is lodged.

You can get more specific by simply continuing to query the body. It's easy, and gets even easier with practice.

Don't discount your own ability to discern where the emotion is trapped. If you simply listen to your intuition for a moment about the location of the trapped emotion, an impression may come into your mind. Check that location first, and you will be surprised at how often it is correct, saving you time and effort.

Once you have found the location of the trapped emotion, think about any symptoms that may be present in that part of the body. If there is pain in the area of the trapped emotion, it may suddenly disappear or dissipate when it is released.

Remembering the Trapped Emotion

Sometimes, you will still not have any idea what event led to the creation of a trapped emotion. Quite often, trapped emotions can be created by circumstances that are quickly forgotten.

Say for example, that one day everything just seemed to go wrong. Perhaps you went to dinner before seeing a show, and the service was terrible. You knew you were going to be late for the show, and you became upset. When the bill finally arrived, your credit card was maxed out, and you chose to feel very angry or humiliated, or both. We can become pretty upset at times when things aren't going our way. The intense emotions we may be feeling on an occasion like this may leave us with a trapped emotion or two. But a year later, you may be hard pressed to remember this event, particularly if you chose not to dwell on the bad experience. If a number of years have gone by, the trapped emotion will still be there, but consciously recalling the event may now become very difficult.

Sometimes trapped emotions are created during an event that was transitory in nature, and the event itself is lost forever to your conscious memory.

Even if you don't remember immediately what a given trapped emotion was about, my experience has been that approximately 50% of the time you will remember within the next couple of days. Typically, the following day or during the night, you will be doing something totally unrelated, when the event will suddenly pop into your mind. You will remember what happened, because your subconscious mind was searching, working overtime trying to figure it out and dredge it up out of your memory bank.

There is no limit to how many times you can ask, "Do we need to know more about this trapped emotion?" Once you get a no answer, you know everything you need to know about it and you can release it.

Whether or not you actually remember what occurred and what created your trapped emotion is not critical to the releasing of the emotional energy. It can be interesting to figure it out, and there may even be some insight to be gained by doing so, but identifying which emotion is trapped and bringing it to conscious awareness is all that is necessary before releasing it. The next step will tell you exactly *how* to release it.

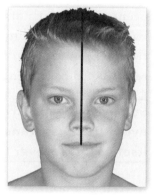

The Governing Meridian

Releasing an Emotion from Yourself

To release a trapped emotion from yourself, place your magnet between your eyebrows on your skin. While you continue to breathe (don't hold your breath) roll or slide the magnet up the middle of your forehead, over the top of your head, and down the back of your neck as far as you can comfortably reach, three times.

You can run your magnet over any part of the Governing Meridian with the intention of releasing the trapped energy that is in your body. If you have "big hair" and you can't go over your hair without messing it up, just use your magnet on your forehead as far as you can. It's that easy. Just remember to do it three times, and to stay focused on your intention to let the trapped emotion go.

Releasing an Emotion from Another Person

To release a trapped emotion from another person, place your magnet on their back at the base of their neck. Instruct your partner to continue to breathe in and

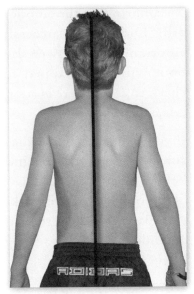

The Governing Meridian

out while you roll or slide the magnet from the base of their neck to their low back or just beyond, three times. Each time you reach the bottom of a stroke, lift the magnet off their back and replace it at the base of the neck.

Each stroke transfers magnetic energy into the Governing Meridian. This magnetic energy magnifies and carries your intention into all the other meridians, filling the body with that intention and thought. The result is that within three strokes, the trapped emotion is released, forever. It's just that simple.

Confirming the Release

To confirm that the emotion has been released, simply ask, "Did (I) we successfully release that trapped emotion?" The answer should be yes. If so, you are done with that trapped emotion, and you can now check to see if there is another trapped emotion to be released, if you wish.

If your test shows that the emotion was not released, simply reapply the magnetic energy three times as before. But this time, have a little more love in your heart for who you are working on, whether yourself or your partner, believe that you can release this emotion, and allow yourself to feel gratitude to God that it is being released.

Remember that all things are accomplished by faith and belief, and if you have a little faith, you'll see great things happen.

Remember the words of Jesus:

> *"...verily I say unto you, If ye have faith as a grain of mustard seed, ye shall say unto this mountain, Remove hence to yonder place; and it shall remove; and nothing shall be impossible unto you." (Matt: 17-20)*

It's Permanent

One of the most beautiful aspects of the Emotion Code is that trapped emotions, once released, are gone forever. In all the years that we have worked with patients in practice and at seminars, we have never seen a trapped emotion that was released ever return.

On the other hand, it is possible for people to have more than one occurrence of a particular emotion lodged in their body. In this case, you might release the same emotion from your subject several times, but each emotion will be a separate and distinct trapped energy, usually resulting from different emotional events in their past. It's also possible for a person to have several distinctly different emotions that all became trapped from the same event.

Dealing With Specific Issues

If you are struggling with a specific problem in your life, it's important to determine if trapped emotions may be playing an unseen role.

You might suspect that you have a trapped emotion, but it doesn't show up when you ask the general question, "Do I have a trapped emotion that I can release now?" Trapped emotions sometimes need to be addressed more directly for them to unveil themselves.

Here are some examples of common problems, along with ways to ask. This list could go on and on, but this will give you an idea of how you can ask about your own specific problems.

"Do I have a trapped emotion that is preventing me from losing weight?"

"Is there a trapped emotion that is causing inflammation in my tissues?"

"Do I have a trapped emotion that is blocking me from making more money?"

"Is there a trapped emotion that is preventing me from selling more widgets?"

"Is there a trapped emotion that is contributing to my (back, neck, shoulder, knee, etc.) pain?

"Do I have a trapped emotion that is causing me to be (depressed, short-tempered, angry, etc.)?"

"Do I have a trapped emotion about my (husband, wife, son, daughter, boss, etc.)?"

"Is there a trapped emotion that is interfering with the achievement of my goals?"

"Is there a trapped emotion that is making it more difficult for me to quit (drinking, smoking, using drugs, pornography, etc.)?"

"Do I have a trapped emotion about (name specific event)?"

If the answer to a direct question like these is yes, the subconscious mind has identified the emotion. You would then continue by asking which column this trapped emotion is in, following the process as I have outlined previously in this chapter, and as shown on the flowchart on page 222.

Remember that there may be more than one emotion contributing to any given issue. In addition, trapped emotions will often come off in layers. If you release a trapped emotion that has to do with a specific issue today, another emotion about that same issue may not show up until later. If you are attempting to overcome a specific issue, it's a good idea to recheck that issue for trapped emotions from time to time.

Nested Emotions

It's not unusual to find several trapped emotions lodged together in a particular area of the body, a phenomenon I refer to as "Nesting." You will sometimes find a significant level of discomfort in your subject when nesting is going on. Having multiple trapped emotions in one area seems to create a greater level of tissue distortion and pain. It is interesting to observe that as nesting trapped emotions are discovered and released using the Emotion Code, the level of discomfort often diminishes noticeably as each one is released. For stories that illustrate nesting, see "Jean's Painful Ovary" on page 73, and "Jack's Tennis Elbow" on page 75.

Processing the Release

As the mindbody processes the emotion that has been released, symptoms of this processing can arise. Once a trapped emotion has been brought to the awareness of the conscious mind, and has been released magnetically as described, at that point a healing process begins.

During this healing process a person may experience echoes of the emotion that has been released. It is not unusual for people to feel a bit emotionally up and down during this period of time.

The body will usually be willing to release at least one emotion before wanting to take time out to process. On the other hand, sometimes the body will release one emotion after another, and do the processing for a group of emotions simultaneously. Remember to trust the wisdom of the body implicitly, and never force it, but be gentle with the body, allowing it the time it needs to process and heal.

If after releasing a trapped emotion, the body will not release another, you can ask when it will be ready to release the next one, by asking "Will I (you) be able to release another trapped emotion _____?" filling in the blank with words like "in 10 minutes", "in 2 hours", "this afternoon", "tomorrow", and so on. If processing is called for, it typically lasts from a few hours to a few days.

Be Aware of Processing Ups and Downs

It's very important to let the person you are working with know that they may experience some slight emotional ups and downs from processing the release of a trapped emotion. If you let them know about this possibility in advance, and it actually occurs, it is expected. If some noticeable processing *does* occur, such as crying or vivid dreams, and you haven't told them that they might experience it, they may end up thinking that the release of their trapped emotion has made them worse, not better.

Processing takes place every time a trapped emotion is released, but noticeable ups and downs occur about 30% of the time. Often the mind-body is capable of processing the release of a trapped emotion without breaking stride; it is a multi-tasking computer, after all. But sometimes, it just takes some time for the mind-body to heal from a trapped emotion, and to get a handle on this new state of affairs.

While a person is processing the release of one or more trapped emotions, they are not restricted in any way from their normal activities.

Prenatal Trapped Emotions

Sometimes you will find that a trapped emotion did not occur at any age from birth onward. Trapped emotions can also occur in the womb. In this case, you can ask:

"Did this emotion become trapped in the womb?"

"Did this emotion become trapped during the 1st trimester?"

"Did this emotion become trapped during the 2nd trimester?"

"Did this emotion become trapped during the 3rd trimester?"

In my experience, prenatal trapped emotions usually develop during the third trimester, and will usually be emotions that the subject's mother was experiencing.

In other words, let's say a woman is in her second or third trimester of pregnancy, and is experiencing the emotion of grief. Her whole being is vibrating with this emotional energy, and the infant begins to resonate with that emotion. As a result, the fetus may get a trapped emotion from its mother.

I have never seen an occasion where a trapped emotion was created by the fetus itself, but whether the emotion was generated by the fetus or by the mother's body doesn't matter. It can be released the same way in either case, by applying the magnet three times to the Governing Meridian as previously described.

Inherited Trapped Emotions

In the same way that you can inherit your eye color or the shape of your nose from your father and mother and other ancestors, you can also inherit trapped emotions from them. An *inherited* trapped emotion is different from a *prenatal* trapped emotion, or from any other type of trapped emotion.

In the case of an inherited emotion, you actually receive the energy of the emotion at the moment of conception from the sperm or the egg.

When the sperm and egg unite, one of them is already carrying an extra passenger in the form of some emotional energy. The now-fertilized egg begins the process of division, and everything that exists in the original egg is now duplicated. As the fertilized egg divides this excess emotional energy is duplicated as well.

You can certainly ask "Is there an inherited emotion that we can release now?" to uncover the existence of this type of trapped energy. But most often, you will stumble across inherited emotions while you are on the trail of what you think is a regular trapped emotion.

How Inherited Emotions are Uncovered

Our experience is that the mind-body will lead you to the correct column and row that an inherited emotion is in, but will not give you a yes answer on any of the five emotions that are listed in that cell, unless and until you preface the emotion with the word *inherited*.

For example, say you have identified that the trapped emotion you are trying to release is in column B row 2. You have tested each of the emotions listed in that cell, but the response is no for each emotion. If this occurs, simply ask "Is this an inherited trapped emotion?" If you receive a yes answer in response, simply go through the emotions again by asking "Is this inherited _____ _____?" filling in the blank with each emotion listed until you find the correct inherited emotion.

Once you have identified the inherited emotion, you might want to determine which parent the subject received this trapped emotion from. To go even deeper, you might ask if this inherited emotion came from a grandparent or a great grandparent, etc. Typically, however, you will find that most inherited trapped emotions will have come from a father, mother or grandparents.

My daughter Natalie was working on me remotely a couple of years ago and found an inherited trapped emotion of hopelessness. When she determined that this emotion dated back 22 generations to an Irish grandmother of mine on my father's side, Natalie suddenly felt the presence of this very woman by her side; she could feel how desperate she was to have this emotion released from her posterity, and at the same time she could feel how grateful she was that this work was being done. I knew the moment this energy was released, because a background feeling of hopelessness that had been there all my life was suddenly gone. I never really knew that it was there, until the moment it was gone!

When an inherited trapped emotion is released, it is released from all the ancestors that passed the emotional energy down the line, no matter how many generations back that may be. This is truly one of the most powerful aspects of The Emotion Code! I recommend that you hold a clear intention to release the inherited trapped emotion from every soul that is holding this energy, whether living or dead, since it is possible that the person you are working on may have passed this energy to their children. When you are finished, you can muscle test to see if the emotion was released from not only the subject, but from anyone else who may have inherited this energy.

Releasing an Inherited Emotion from Yourself

To release an inherited trapped emotion from yourself, place your magnet between your eyebrows on your skin and follow the procedure already described for releasing a non-inherited trapped emotion. The difference is simply that while you continue to breathe (don't hold your breath) roll or slide the magnet up the middle of your forehead, over the top of your head, and down the back of your neck as far as you can comfortably reach, TEN times instead of only three times.

Releasing an Inherited Emotion from Another

To release an inherited trapped emotion from another person, place your magnet on their back at the base of their neck. Instruct your partner to continue to breathe in and out while you roll or slide the magnet from the base of their neck to their low back or just beyond, TEN times instead of three times. Each time you reach the bottom of a stroke, lift the magnet off their back and replace it at the base of the neck.

Pre-Conception Trapped Emotions

On rare occasions, I have discovered trapped emotions that actually occurred prior to conception, and I am not referring to inherited emotions. I believe that prior to conception we existed as conscious entities, but we were without physical bodies. Instead, we existed as spirit-beings. We could think for ourselves, and we were aware of our coming journey to earth.

Most pre-conception trapped emotions are about our impending sojourn on earth.

It seems that sometimes, even though we may rejoice in our opportunity to come to the earth, we become frightened or dismayed by the journey ahead of us. To leave that place of beauty and love, to come here to this earth, with all its trouble, violence, and war might make even the stoutest heart wilt. Sometimes pre-conception trapped emotions have to do with some sort of grief or sadness about leaving our heavenly home. But I have also seen cases where trapped emotions were created by relationship problems from long ago. Preconception trapped emotions are somewhat unusual, but I have seen them, and you probably will, too. And although they are unusual and can often be quite powerful, they are released like other trapped emotions, with three swipes of the magnet, once they are brought to conscious awareness.

As you use the Emotion Code to help yourself and others, you will find joy in seeing the progress that a person can make as they shed their burdens one by one. You will see lives changed, people healed, and hearts connected.

Don't give up! It takes some time to become proficient at the Emotion Code. Trust in your own healing abilities. It is well worth the effort. Believe and be grateful to God that you can do this, and the outcome will be your reward for believing.

In the next chapter you will learn how trapped emotions can create a wall around your heart, blocking your ability to give and receive love.

For your convenience, if you'd like to download a fully printable copy of the two following pages, simply visit my website at:

HealersLibrary.com/flowcharts

The Emotion Code™ Flowchart

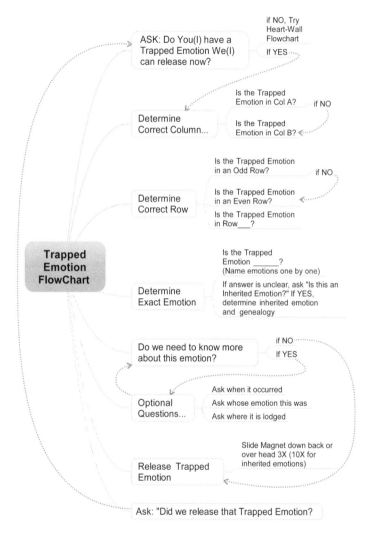

Follow this flowchart and the Chart of Emotions on the right to release trapped emotions.

The Emotion Code™ Chart

	Column A	Column B
Row 1 Heart or Small Intestine	Abandonment Betrayal Forlorn Lost Love Unreceived	Effort Unreceived Heartache Insecurity Overjoy Vulnerability
Row 2 Spleen or Stomach	Anxiety Despair Disgust Nervousness Worry	Failure Helplessness Hopelessness Lack of Control Low Self-Esteem
Row 3 Lung or Colon	Crying Discouragement Rejection Sadness Sorrow	Confusion Defensiveness Grief Self-Abuse Stubborness
Row 4 Liver or Gall Bladder	Anger Bitterness Guilt Hatred Resentment	Depression Frustration Indecisiveness Panic Taken for Granted
Row 5 Kidneys or Bladder	Blaming Dread Fear Horror Peeved	Conflict Creative Insecurity Terror Unsupported Wishy Washy
Row 6 Glands & Sexual Organs	Humiliation Jealousy Longing Lust Overwhelm	Pride Shame Shock Unworthy Worthless

I DON'T WANNA LOOK LIKE SOME KIND OF FOOL-
I DON'T WANNA BREAK MY HEART OVER YOU.
I'M BUILDING A WALL. EVERYDAY IT'S GETTING HIGHER.
THIS TIME I WON'T END UP ANOTHER VICTIM OF LOVE.
I'M GONNA LOCK UP WHAT I'M FEELING INSIDE.
AIN'T NO WAY YOU CAN BREAK DOWN THE DOOR.

- "VICTIM OF LOVE" LYRICS BY THE GROUP ERASURE

7

THE WALLS AROUND OUR HEARTS

Trapped emotions can create a wall around your heart that can block you from living life to the fullest. I received this letter from a wonderful woman, a former patient of mine who had a Heart-Wall, once upon a time...

Living the Fairy Tale

At the time Dr. Nelson cleared my Heart-Wall, I was approximately 51 years old and I had worked at the Walt Disney Company for 22 years. It was a busy, exciting career, filled with travel all over the world and bright, creative people. I had a wonderful family and many close friendships. I had never been married. I wasn't against marriage nor was I dying to get married. It wasn't an issue. My life was full.

Later that year, two of my friends were planning a trip to China. They asked me to join them, but I said I was very busy at work. They kept up their encouragement. It was as if an invisible hand was at my back, pushing me in the direction of China. Thinking that if I ever did want to go to China, I may as well go, I went.

Travel in China was somewhat restricted at the time, so we went with a group. There was a wonderful gentleman on the trip, an attorney who had been divorced for seven years. He lived in Newport Beach, about 40 miles from my home up the California coast. We got to know each other in a very unassuming way during our tour of China.

On the airplane trip home, we sat together and he asked me out for the following weekend. We dated for a year. He popped the question on Thanksgiving Day and we were married six months later. I was age 53.

As I reflect back on the time after my Heart-Wall cleared, I realize things weren't the same. I began to open myself to the idea of having someone in my life "to have and to hold" and to care for as he would care for me. It happened on the feeling level. Finding someone to share my life with just felt like the next step. There was a new readiness that I *hadn't felt before. It must have been the removal of that invisible wall — that I had not even known was there — that allowed me to let this wonderful man in.*

So for all of you who think women cannot marry after "a certain age," get your Heart-Wall cleared, stay open to the possibilities life has to offer and remember my story. We are now approaching our 5th anniversary, have just moved into our new home on the California Coast overlooking the ocean and Catalina Island and are living the fairy tale.

Thank you, Dr. Nelson.

Lynn R., California

The Heart-Brain

Your heart generates 60 to 1000 times more power and electromagnetic energy than your brain, easily making it the most powerful organ in your body. When you were in the womb, your heart was formed first, before your brain. Your heart beats about 100,000 times a day, 40 million times a year, and if its connection to your brain were severed, it would keep right on beating.

Your heart is the core of your being, the core of who you really are.

New research shows that your heart is much more than a mere pump. In the 1970s, scientists learned that the heart has an elaborate nervous system, a discovery that has led to the creation of a new branch of medicine known as neurocardiology. The fact is, we all have *two* brains. Much to these scientists' surprise, they discovered that the brains in our heads are *obeying* messages sent by "the brains in our hearts."

Your heart is constantly sending out information to your body. Every beat carries critical messages that affect your emotional and physical health.

When you feel love toward someone, you are actually sending out a powerful electromagnetic signal to them, using the heart brain.

Medical research experiments have repeatedly shown that there are measurable positive effects on the body when we feel love and appreciation toward someone else. The same beneficial affect occurs in your own body when you are on the receiving end – when love and appreciation are being broadcast toward you.[1]

Scientists have discovered that the electromagnetic signals radiating from your heart are actually detectable in the brain waves of another person. This phenomenon is strongest when two people are touching or are in close proximity but is measurable at a distance as well.[2]

1 Rollin McCraty, Ph.D., edited by P. J. Rosch and M. S. Markov. "The Energetic Heart: Bioelectromagnetic Communication Within and Between People", *Clinical Applications of Bioelectromagnetic Medicine*, (2004), 541-562.

2 R. McCraty, M. Atkinson and W. Tiller, *The Role of Physiological Coherence in the Detection and Measurement of Cardiac Energy Exchange Between People* (Proceedings of the Tenth International Montreux Congress on Stress, Montreux, Switzerland, 1999).

For several decades, medical science has had the remarkable ability to transplant organs from one person's body to another. But remember the story of the World War II veteran and his blood cells. If a person's individual cells keep their connection so strongly no matter where they are, think what a connection an entire organ must retain! We've all heard stories about transplant recipients who suddenly take an interest in a certain sport, or who have an unexplained craving for their donor's favorite food. Heart transplant patients have reported these symptoms from the beginning, but doctors have had no way to understand it, so they attributed it to the patients' imaginations.

Try telling that to the transplant patient who has never liked hot dogs or baseball, but who now can't get enough of them since he received the heart of an avid White Sox fan. Or the woman who can't keep from crying every time she hears a certain song, a song which meant nothing to her before her transplant.

The heart has its own unique intelligence. It can think, feel and remember.

There is now considerable evidence that the heart contains memories and feelings. A large number of heart transplant recipients have reported new food and drink preferences and cravings, as well as handwriting changes, musical preferences, and memories that don't seem to be their own.[3]

3 Mindshock: Transplanting Memories. Channel4.com, Belfast, Northern Ireland. http://video.google.com/videoplay?docid=-2219468990718192402

The Discovery of the Heart-Wall

Have you ever felt that you needed to "put up a wall" to protect yourself in a negative situation? It appears that this common phrase has a basis in reality. We call this phenomenon the "Heart-Wall", and here is how we were led to discover it.

In March of 1998, my wife Jean and I were in Portland, Oregon, attending a conference on magnetic healing where I was one of the guest speakers.

Early one morning, she woke me to say she'd had a powerful dream. She felt strongly that her dream had a deep meaning, and that it had something to do with her own health.

In her dream, Jean saw a stainless steel order wheel like those found in restaurants and diners. She explained that the wheel had three orders clipped to it. She understood intuitively that each order represented a different issue having to do with her health.

Her subconscious mind knew the meaning of this dream, so I began muscle testing her, asking questions about the orders attached to the wheel. We quickly determined the meaning of the first two health issues. When I turned my attention to the third order on the wheel, something completely unexpected happened.

Suddenly I had a waking vision.

I could see very clearly in my mind's eye a beautiful, highly polished hardwood floor. Along with this vision came the understanding that Jean's *heart* was *under* this floor!

This made no logical sense, but the image of this gleaming floor, and the perception that her heart was under it, were very persistent and clear. I determined to figure out what it all meant, if I could. I told Jean what I was seeing, and asked her if she had any insight into what this meant.

"Well, last night I wasn't feeling all that well, and Lana told me that she sensed there was some kind of energy over my heart. I wonder if that is what she was picking up." My sister-in-law Lana is a Reiki Master, and a very gifted and intuitive healer. "I really don't know what it means."

Fascinated, we began muscle testing to find out more about this hardwood flood.

"First, let's find out how thick this floor is," I said. "Is it one plank thick?"

Her arm was strong. The answer was "Yes."

"Is it two planks thick?" "Yes."

"It is three planks thick?" "Yes."

Patiently, we went up by the numbers – five planks, ten planks, twenty, fifty, 100, 200 ... Before long, I began asking about the thickness in feet.

"Is this floor 100 feet thick?" "Yes."

"Is it 500 feet thick?" "Yes."

And on it went — 1000 feet, 2000 feet, 3000 feet, 4000 … "Is it 5000 feet thick?" "Yes."

"Is this floor a mile thick?" "Yes."

"Is it two miles, three miles, four miles thick?" "Yes, yes, yes."

"Is this floor five miles thick?" "Yes."

"Is this floor six miles thick?" "No."

This was quite strange, and we couldn't imagine what it meant. I was certain that it had some significant meaning, so I continued testing. It quickly became apparent that the hardwood floor I could see so clearly in my mind was exactly five miles thick. I had never had a waking vision like this before, yet the answers we were getting were very clear.

Three things were certain. I could see the floor vividly in my mind. I knew that in some symbolic way my wife's heart was underneath this floor. The floor was very thick, five miles thick to be exact. What in the world could this possibly mean?

I asked, "Is there a wall around your heart?" "Yes."

"Is this wall five miles thick?" "Yes."

"Is it made of wood?" "Yes."

What exactly was this that we were in the process of discovering? Was it something of consequence?

Quieting my mind for a moment led me to ask another question. "Is this wall made up of trapped emotions?"

Her arm was strong. The answer was "Yes."

Suddenly the symbolic meaning became clear to me. I knew how vulnerable the human heart is to being hurt. I also knew Jean's past.

Jean had been a sensitive and shy little girl. She had grown up in an imperfect, dysfunctional household like many of us do. While she has some wonderful memories, and while she loved her parents and siblings and knew they loved her, she didn't feel safe emotionally.

She could never predict what the emotional tone in her home might be from one moment to the next. Anger and harsh words frequently and suddenly erupted over things that should have been inconsequential. She and other family members would find themselves "walking on eggshells" at times like these. She never knew when she or someone else in the family might be lashed out at or blamed for something.

Protecting the Core of You

People deal with uncomfortable situations such as these in many ways. Some attack, some retreat, and some hide. But usually, we feel the need to defend and shield ourselves from being hurt.

Your heart is the core of your being. Your subconscious mind knows that it must protect your heart; it must protect your delicate core in any way it can.

Words like "heartache" and "heartbreak" are so-called because of the peculiar physical sensation that occurs in the heart under strong emotional strain. Nearly everyone has felt this sensation at one point or another.

Trapped emotions have substance. They consist of energy, just like everything else. When trapped emotions are created, they must reside somewhere in your body, and sometimes they will lodge in and around your heart.

Your subconscious mind – which knows no limitations – will sometimes use the energy of these trapped emotions to create a barrier or shield around your heart. Literally, it creates a wall of energy around your heart, to protect it.

At first, I puzzled over this process until I realized that the subconscious mind most likely follows certain rules. For example, it is not possible to create a wall out of nothing. In the world in which we live, all things around us are made of energy, and I believe the subconscious mind understands this concept implicitly. All walls that exist in the physical world around us, regardless of the chosen building material, are ultimately made of energy. The Heart-Wall, created by the subconscious mind, is also made of energy. It just happens to be made of a specific sort of energy, the energy of trapped emotions.

I believe that to the subconscious mind, the Heart-Wall is as real as the chair you are sitting in. The Heart-Wall exists, it's just on a slightly different plane of reality than the world we can see with our physical eyes. Does that make the Heart-Wall any less real? I don't think so. Remember that we cannot see ultraviolet light or indeed, the vast majority of the electromagnetic spectrum, yet no one disputes its reality.

When I asked Jean's body if we could release the trapped emotions that were making up this wall around her heart, the answer was "Yes."

Gradually, her body was willing to release these emotions. We found that the procedure for releasing emotions from the Heart-Wall was the same as for releasing any other trapped emotion. The only difference was that we had to ask specifically if we could release an emotion "from her Heart-Wall" in order to gain access to those emotions.

Each time we released a trapped emotion from Jean's Heart-Wall, I would ask if we could release another emotion. Sometimes her body would allow us to clear more than one emotion in a single session, but often the answer was "No."

It wasn't surprising that her body needed a certain amount of time to process each of her emotions as they were released, so we patiently waited between sessions. We found that we were able to release a different trapped emotion roughly every other day until they were all gone, and Jean no longer had a Heart-Wall.

The Creation of Her Heart-Wall

Jean had learned to protect her feelings from childhood. She retreated to safety inside of herself, shutting down her positive feelings, and avoiding connection with those that she felt vulnerable toward. When there were volatile episodes in her home, she chose to feel fear, resentment and other negative emotions, some of which she expressed, but many that she internalized. Some of these feelings were never fully processed, and they became trapped energies in her body.

While she was consciously doing her best to deal with life, at the same time her subconscious was building a wall, an ultimate protection against her heart being injured again.

Her subconscious mind chose an imaginary wooden floor for her wall, specifically the hardwood that is walked upon. Do you see the symbolism there? The room she grew up in had a hardwood floor, as did much of her house back then, so it was a familiar sight. Her subconscious mind created her Heart-Wall at an early age, but it wasn't completed for many years.

Each new trapped emotion gave her wall additional thickness and strength, until it was many thousands of feet thick.

As we released the emotions from her Heart-Wall, we found that the thickness of the wall decreased. We could never predict how much of a decrease in thickness might result with the release of a trapped emotion. Some trapped emotions would result in a large decrease in thickness, some in a little.

When the last trapped emotion was released, something very interesting happened that helped Jean move beyond her past and the way that she perceived herself.

Getting Reconnected Again

While Jean's Heart-Wall protected her heart from damage and hurt, this protection came at a cost.

Having a Heart-Wall left her feeling numb and somewhat isolated. She felt disconnected from others. She wanted to have close friends, and she tried many times, but something was always in the way. She was well-liked, but she found it hard to be at ease with people. She had many associations, but few close friends. In social gatherings, even with people she had known for many years, she invariably felt that she was on the outside looking in, and she was never able to feel like she truly belonged.

When the last trapped emotion was finally released, and her Heart-Wall was gone, there was a profound shift.

"For the first time in my life, I'm not on the outside anymore," she told me. "I've longed to feel this way my whole life. Now I know what it feels like to be part of a circle of friends, part of a group. It's a very different feeling than I've ever had before, and it feels wonderful and right."

Since that day, these feeling have stayed with her, and have helped her to grow in many ways. We've since discovered that releasing someone's Heart-Wall is often followed by a profound experience of connection with other people.

Much of our personal and spiritual growth comes out of our love and interaction with others. The more open our hearts are, the stronger will be our connection to one another. The more connected we are, the more we can give and receive love, and the stronger and richer our lives will become.

I am so grateful for Jean and her dream that day. Without her, the Heart-Wall might still be completely unknown.

When we began to test other people for Heart-Walls, we found that they are a very common problem. Our experience is that eight out of ten people have one. Chances are, you do, too.

Joanne's Bad Marriage

One of the first people we tested for a Heart-Wall was a woman named Joanne. She had been married for twenty-two years and had five children. Her husband was mentally and verbally abusive. He had created such a toxic experience in their home that the rest of the family wondered why she chose to stay in such a bad marriage year after year.

Like most women in her position, Joanne had endured the marriage by creating a Heart-Wall that helped insulate her tender heart from her husband's abusive verbal and emotional assaults.

I suspected that Joanne had a Heart-Wall, and her body responded "Yes" when I asked if she did. Next I wondered what her Heart-Wall might be made of. Were all Heart-Walls made of wood? I didn't know, but when I asked that question, her body said "No."

Not wood. Well, how about some kind of metal? The answer was "Yes", some kind of metal.

"Is the metal iron?" I asked, trying to narrow it down. "No."

"Is it steel?" I asked. "No."

I tried titanium, aluminum, copper and all the other kinds of metal I had ever heard of, but the answer was always "No."

So I approached from a different angle. "Is this metal harder than iron?" "Yes."

"Is this metal harder than steel?" Again, "Yes."

As I continued this line of questioning, it gradually became apparent that the metal was harder than all the metals I could name. Feeling a bit exasperated, I asked, "Is your Heart-Wall made of metal that is harder than any metal that actually exists on earth? "Her answer was definitive: "Yes."

Wait a minute. What? How could her Heart-Wall be made of a metal that was harder than any metal that existed on earth?

Something Out of This World

I was so caught up in my concrete questions that I'd forgotten one very important fact.

The Heart-Wall is a creation of the subconscious mind – where literally anything is possible.

This wall is not physically made of any materials except the energy of a certain number of trapped emotions. It may not be "real" to us, but I believe that to the subconscious mind, although it is imaginary, it is also as real as anything else that exists in the world.

Its reality in the body is a very powerful one. That reality affects the systems of the body, just as our thoughts do. It has a direct influence on our health. But remember, the Heart-Wall is an imaginary construct – it can be made of literally anything at all.

Two years after Joanne was married, the abuse began. Her highest value was to keep her marriage together, so she stayed put.

Joanne had grown up in an idyllic and serene home, where she was cherished. According to Joanne, she could not remember her parents ever fighting, and the number of times that angry words were spoken could be counted on the fingers of one hand.

As the abuse increased in her marriage, her subconscious mind searched desperately for protection. Trapped emotions were being formed, so the raw materials were there to build a wall, but what kind of material would her subconscious mind consider to be tough enough to protect her heart from Nick's abuse?

It is said that the subconscious mind does not distinguish between what we perceive to be either "reality" or "non-reality." For example, if you see a movie that is very frightening, your subconscious mind doesn't "know" that you are not actually experiencing the celluloid-reality of the movie. Sure enough, your heart will pound, your palms will sweat, and your biochemical reactions will be just the same. Adrenalin will course through your veins, and all the reactions that occur in a fight or flight situation will be the same as if your viewed reality is, indeed, reality itself.

Essentially, the subconscious mind treats everything that comes into it from your conscious mind as reality, whether it is or not. Which brings us back to Joanne, who has a Heart-Wall made of metal, but a certain kind of metal, stronger than any metal that exists on earth.

At some point, long ago, Joanne had seen an alien spaceship on a science fiction show. The Army fired missiles at it. When the smoke cleared, it was still there. They shot cannons at it – to no effect. They even launched a nuclear warhead at this alien spacecraft, but when the smoke cleared, it was still there. The scientists were stunned; the spacecraft was made of an entirely unknown substance, a metal that did not exist on earth, one that was apparently indestructible.

"Yes!" Her subconscious mind said, "That's exactly what I need!" And this alien, make believe metal from an old sci-fi movie became her Heart-Wall construction material.

So Joanne had a Heart-Wall made of indestructible metal from an alien spacecraft. What better way to protect her heart? Remember, the Heart-Wall is from the deep imagination, from the subconscious mind of the person who unconsciously creates it.

Once we'd found out what it was made of at the metaphorical level, we began to release the trapped emotions that had been organized into this wall around Joanne's heart.

Because she was still in this marriage with her abusive husband, we realized that her Heart-Wall had probably been a very important factor in her remaining married to Nick.

It had protected her heart all these years. Was removing the Heart-Wall the right thing to do? Was it the right thing for Joanne, at this point in her life? Her body had created the Heart-Wall for a reason, but there is always a price that you pay when you have a Heart-Wall, that price mainly being a diminished ability to feel.

We decided that the only safe route would be to ask her subconscious mind if it was okay to begin releasing these trapped emotions that were making up her Heart-Wall.

"Can we release a trapped emotion from your Heart-Wall now?" I asked.

Her body said "Yes." It was okay to begin getting rid of these trapped emotions that were making up her Heart-Wall. In fact, Joanne's body wanted them gone! So we began to clear them out, finding them one at a time through muscle testing.

Each time we would release a trapped emotion, we would re-check the thickness of the Heart-Wall, which we had initially found to be seven feet thick.

"Is the Heart-Wall still seven feet thick?" "No," her body responded.

"Is it six feet thick?" "Yes."

Again, with every trapped emotion we released, her Heart-Wall became thinner. The distance by which the

Heart-Wall thickness diminished varied, depending on the emotion. Sometimes one released emotion would reduce the Heart-Wall by an entire foot. Other times, a released emotion would make less difference, resulting in a six-inch change or less. In Joanne's case, there was no waiting period between releasing one emotion and the next; her subconscious mind was ready to release them all in a row, just as fast as we could find them and let them go.

Connecting the Dots

As we identified each trapped emotion, I also asked when that specific trapped emotion had become trapped. Asking that question helped Joanne connect the trapped emotions to specific events in her life that had caused her so much pain. We found that she did not have a Heart-Wall until the second year of her marriage, when things really started to become difficult.

As we traced back the origins of the individual trapped emotions, it was easy to see why Joanne had needed a Heart-Wall that was indestructible. One of her trapped emotions was from the time her husband had held a gun to his head and threatened to kill himself in front of her. Another trapped emotion was from the time that he fell into a fit of rage over her religious practices and literally burned her Bible in front of her. There were nine different emotions that had become trapped in her body, each of them having to do with some extreme experience with her husband, Nick.

Feeling Again With Her Heart

It took about thirty minutes to release all nine of these emotions and completely clear Joanne's Heart-Wall. When her body indicated that the Heart-Wall was gone, Joanne smiled quietly.

"How are you feeling?" I asked her.

"A little dazed," she said. "But good..." Then she went back home to Nick.

For twenty-two years, Joanne had an impenetrable wall around her heart. Now that the wall was gone, suddenly, she was able to feel in her heart all the barbs, all the meanness and all the venom that Nick heaped on her, from the moment she walked in the door.

For the first time in many years, she was really *feeling* what was going on in her relationship with Nick. Her Heart-Wall had been shielding her from the full force of his cruelty. Now that she could experience it for what it really was, without the protective wall, she couldn't believe she'd stayed with him for so long. Who could tolerate this kind of abuse? And why should she put up with it anymore? Within two weeks she had left Nick for good, and filed for divorce.

Like so many of our body's defenses, a Heart-Wall can be an invaluable safety measure in the short-term.

When something overwhelming happens, an emergency action can save your life.

If you're being bombed, it's a good idea to hide in a bunker. But you wouldn't want to live there. If you did, you'd miss out on the joys and wonders of life.

The same is true with a Heart-Wall. No matter how important it was to your life at the time it was created, you will be able to live a happier, more connected life as soon as you can tear it down. Sometimes, it can make the difference between living a life of disappointment and living happily ever after.

Miranda and the Old Boyfriend

Miranda is a perfect example of how a Heart-Wall can interfere with your love life. She was an attractive 38-year-old nurse who came to me suffering from neck pain. During the course of the examination, she mentioned that she had not dated anyone in years and had no interest in having any kind of a relationship with men anymore. When I tested her, I was not surprised to find that she had a Heart-Wall.

Eight years before, Miranda's heart had been broken in a relationship with a man she had deeply loved. In an effort to protect her heart from experiencing that kind of pain and injury again, her subconscious mind had created a Heart-Wall.

In Miranda's case, three lingering emotions had been trapped in her body for all those years, blocking her from experiencing a loving relationship. She had no idea that these trapped emotions were the major underlying cause of the pain she was experiencing in her neck as well. Her neck pain had been going on for some time, and was considered chronic and even a bit mysterious by the other doctors she had consulted, as nothing seemed to relieve it.

One by one, we cleared each of these emotions. At the end, I asked her body if the Heart-Wall had finally been released. Her body said that it was completely gone.

I didn't see Miranda again for about three months. When I did, she looked incredibly happy. I asked her what had changed and she excitedly said, "Everything!" She reported that her neck pain was long gone. But there was even better news than that.

"Right after I saw you last," she said, "I ran into my childhood sweetheart. I hadn't seen him since elementary school. But it turned out, he'd been living right around the corner from me — less than a block away — for almost eight years. We started dating and something really sparked between us. We're in love! I think he's going to ask me to marry him."

The woman who had come into my office complaining of neck pain and swearing off men was gone for good. She was like a completely new person.

"Thank you so much for helping me," Miranda said. "If you hadn't released my Heart-Wall, I honestly don't think this would have happened. I was too closed-off before."

When trapped emotions and Heart-Walls are released, people sometimes say it's like they can finally feel again. They can give and receive love freely for the first time in a long time. In that state, very interesting and wonderful things can happen.

How We Are Meant to Live

This is how we're meant to live. We're meant to live vibrant, healthy lives, filled with love and joy. Of all the emotions, love is the most pure and has the highest vibration. Love, that most powerful and most popular of all the emotions, is both *generated* by the heart and *received* by the heart.

When you have a Heart-Wall, you are not able to give love as well as you might, because that love energy that is in your heart cannot get out as well.

At the same time, love that is being radiated toward you by other people is blocked to some degree.

As a result, you can go through your life somewhat insulated from others, because of the emotional traumas you've been through and the subconscious wall that literally exists around your heart. The traumas were genuine enough and there is no doubt that they caused more pain than your body thought it could stand to feel again — that's why the Heart-Wall made perfect sense at the time. But until you take it down, you'll be trapped behind it to some degree, less able to reach out and connect with people, even the people you love most.

People's lives and the lives of their children and their families have been completely transformed when their Heart-Walls have been removed.

About thirty percent of the time, the effects of releasing a Heart-Wall are very apparent and immediately noticeable, but most of the time the results are subtle, and the changes in a person's life appear gradually, in ways that they themselves might not immediately recognize.

Paula and Her Angry Son

One day a woman named Paula came to my office with her son, Rick, who was 17 at the time. She told me that Rick was having problems with anger. He was hanging around with the wrong crowd and his grades were abysmal. She was afraid the next step might be drug use, and was looking to me for help. She had heard of our work with trapped emotions and was wondering if some of her son's anger might be due to them.

I tested this very silent and angry young man and found that he had a Heart-Wall. When I tested his mother, I wasn't too surprised to find that she had a Heart-Wall as well.

It quickly became apparent that Rick wasn't the only one suffering from anger. His mother was also filled with anger and resentment toward her ex-husband, Rick's father. She had a rather grim expression, and her jaw seemed to be set in a determined, angry clench.

It took 5 different sessions to clear Rick's Heart-Wall, each session taking no more than 10 minutes or so. Sometimes he was able to release two emotions during a session, but most of the time, just one. His Heart-Wall trapped emotions all revolved around his birth father and how he had felt abandoned by him over the last few years. His parent's divorce had been terribly difficult for him. He had trapped emotions of anger, frustration, resentment and feelings of inferiority, among other negative emotions.

As soon as we'd completed the process, Rick started to change. It was amusing to see that even his hairstyle changed. When I first met him, Rick had an orange Mohawk; in his case, an expression of his defiance. Without the need to express anger and resentment anymore, he went back to more ordinary hair. Not only that, but his grades improved by several levels. He had always been a smart boy, but he was blocking his emotions behind a Heart-Wall and the pressure had been building up for a long time.

Before we released his Heart-Wall, feelings of rage would well up inside of Rick when he thought of his father. After we cleared the Heart-Wall, Rick could think about his father — even spend time with him — and be completely okay. Now that his simmering anger was a thing of the past, Rick felt happier and more motivated. When he let go of the Heart-Wall, he got his life back.

I will never forget the last time I saw Rick, and how dramatically transformed he was. I remember him not being able to wipe the smile off his face as he told me about a recent fishing trip with his birth-father, and how much his relationship with him had changed.

Curiously enough, when we cleared his mother's Heart-Wall, she didn't seem to notice any change. About two months after we cleared her Heart-Wall, Paula came back to the office and complained to me, saying "What's going on? Rick is like a completely new person. I hardly recognize him. But I don't feel any different than I felt before!"

I explained that, when a Heart-Wall is removed, it often takes time for changes to be felt and for things to realign in your life.

The body has to go through a healing process once a Heart-Wall is removed, and that can take some time.

It was hard to tell whether she accepted that explanation or not. I think she was disappointed that her own life hadn't changed as dramatically as Rick's. I didn't see either of them for a while and wondered on occasion how they were doing.

Then about a year later, I ran into Paula in a very upscale department store in Orange County. She recognized me and waited to see if I would recognize her. She looked familiar, but I had no idea who she was. As we talked, it dawned on me who she was, but she looked so completely different that I scarcely recognized her. Her face radiated happiness. Her whole demeanor had changed. Since we had last seen each other, she had not only gotten a wonderful job at this store, but had also found a wonderful man, and they were happily married.

As we talked, I found that Rick was continuing to do very well both in school and in life. I reminded her about her Heart-Wall and our conversation of a year before.

"I don't know if having my Heart-Wall cleared had something to do with this or not," she grinned, "but my life is so much better now than it was a year ago I can hardly believe it!"

As I walked away from that encounter, I remembered how deeply angry and unhappy she had been only a year before and I couldn't help but wonder where she would be if we had not cleared her Heart-Wall.

Children and Heart-Walls

It's a sad fact of life on this planet, that children often have Heart-Walls, too.

Think how tender and open a child's heart is when they are little. They are helpless and trusting, and far too often, they are the victims of predatory or abusive adults and sometimes even cruel children. In these cases, Heart-Walls are always found.

Sometimes life is challenging even in wonderful homes and under the best of circumstances. The following letter is from a delightful woman whose son was diagnosed as being clinically depressed. After developing a trapped emotion while witnessing the death of a close friend, a Heart-Wall was formed to keep his poor little heart from entirely breaking.

Nine Years Old, and Depressed

Dear Doctor Nelson,

Several weeks ago I brought my nine-year-old son to see you. He had been exhibiting unusual behavior. He was having difficulty eating, sleeping, and concentrating. He had become angry, negative and pessimistic. School was a nightmare! We tried urging, punishing, rewarding and bribing him to complete his school assignments. When they were finally completed he would not turn them into the teacher. He is a very intelligent boy yet his grades suffered because his assignments were not turned in.

I set up an appointment with his pediatrician to be evaluated. We were then referred to a pediatric neurologist, and then to a psychologist for further review – they concluded that my son was depressed. (Two years ago my son witnessed the drowning of a very close friend and ten months later was whisked away to the funeral of his cousin. Four other relatives were buried within the next six months and I believe these events had a distressing effect on my son. I tried to help him cope with these events, but apparently they were still affecting him.)

When I brought him to see you, he was tested and you determined that he had a "Heart-Wall" causing an emotional imbalance in his body. The MagCreator was used to roll-out each of the negative emotions associated with the Heart-Wall. I do not understand all the scientific aspects of this type of treatment yet I believed I had finally found the answer to the growing problems with my son. After you worked on him he was a little lethargic for a couple of days, but the changes I noticed in his behavior in the weeks that followed were absolutely incredible!

By the end of the first week he was sleeping and eating normally, and was once again happy and enthusiastic. He now completes every homework assignment without any nudging on my part. Our home is much more pleasant — he is helpful, kind and patient. I feel like my sweet little boy has returned!

If skepticism had kept me away from this type of treatment, I would still be parenting a very sad and frustrated little boy with no solution in sight. Instead, I have found a treatment that has literally saved him. Thank you Dr. Nelson for all your help. Your knowledge and expertise in this field and your patience and concern have had a tremendous impact... My heartfelt gratitude to you for all that you have done to heal my son.

Thank you!! - (Name Withheld)

Little Jacob's Heart-Wall

One of the most touching experiences I had with children is told by a young mother named Meisha. Her three year old son, Jacob had developed a Heart-Wall shortly after his birth and the death of his twin brother. I treated him and released his Heart-Wall in one visit, and later she wrote this testimonial for you to read.

Three and a half years ago I gave birth to twin sons. Nine days following birth they contracted a virus, which ultimately attacked their hearts, leaving them in critical condition for two months. Jordan, the eldest twin, passed away due to multiple complications leaving Jacob, who then quickly recovered enough to come home but with continual problems with his heart.

Not only was Jacob left with heart failure, but with a Heart-Wall made from deep, lasting emotions that were manifested in excessive anger, destructiveness, unhappiness, insecurity and aggression. A day or two following treatment my tender hearted son was back. Friends would comment on how happy he appeared. He was helpful and kind, patient and pleasant. His behavior was polar opposite from when his heavy emotions were weighing him down. I know through continued treatments my dear son will be emotionally healed and allowed to live the happy life that he is entitled to.

- Meisha E., Texas

As news of our discovery of the Heart-Wall spread, other practitioners began to come to us for training, although the majority of attendees continued to be lay-people. The following Heart-Wall story was submitted by Gwen Legler, a counselor in Washington State.

The Hated Heart-Wall

I have found that people usually choose a Heart-Wall substance that has a positive memory or image for them. That is why I was so surprised with Pearl's negative reaction to her Heart-Wall made of Rhododendron bushes. She hated rhododendrons and couldn't believe her subconscious chose them. I double-checked, and it was correct. I found it interesting that her body would not let me identify her Heart-Wall until the third visit, and then it would only let me remove a few emotions. It was definitely protecting her from something. I suggested we continue and maybe we would understand why.

By the fifth visit we began to remove more emotions – guilt, heartache, hatred, betrayal, grief, and so on. It soon became apparent that her Heart-Wall was like a storage unit for one particular incident in her life. About 16 years ago she had an extramarital affair for which she felt extreme guilt and self-loathing. Although she stopped and never had another affair and was forgiven by her husband, she couldn't seem to forgive herself and put it behind her. Now we realized her Heart-Wall was a bush she hated because it contained an experience she hated. We cleared the Heart-Wall and she found peace and was able to forgive herself.

- Gwen L., Washington

The Ring Dream

Pat and her husband Jim attended the first seminar that I taught, which was held in San Diego in 1996. I received this letter from them about their experience with a recurring nightmare that was being caused by a Heart-Wall.

I wanted to share my experiences with Heart-Walls with you. Jimmy and I attended a seminar in San

Diego with you, where you explained Heart-Walls, how to find them, and break through them.

My daughter died in 1987, and after a while I began having a recurring nightmare that we called "The Ring Dream." Nancy had loved rings, so I always connected the dream with her. I would wake up hysterical and screaming, clutching my hands looking for my rings. I could never remember what caused the panic, or why it was so important to find my rings.

After we attended your seminar, we decided to check me for a Heart-Wall. Needless to say, we found one! We worked back through the years, clearing the layers of trapped emotions as we went. At two years of age, I had a trapped emotion of abandonment. As I had always been with my family, I did not quite believe what the testing was showing. I told my mother about the Heart-Wall, and the abandonment emotion. She told me that when I was two, she had left me with my grandmother and had gone to stay with my father at an Army camp. My grandmother had said for her to go, that she would take care of me, that I was just a baby and wouldn't miss my mother. It was a story that I had never heard before, but it had left its impression on me when I was 2 years old.

Jimmy and I worked together and cleared all the trapped emotions that were making up my Heart-Wall. What a relief it was to us to discover that the dream stopped, and did not return. While we both felt we learned a lot at your seminar, nothing compared to the joy we felt we received when that horrible dream stopped.

I appreciate the opportunity to share this with you. We have shared this story with other people we have met, but I'm glad to finally be able to tell you about it. Thank you so much for this wonderful program.

- Pat S., Louisiana

Finding and Releasing the Heart-Wall

Now let's talk about how you can actually determine if a person has a Heart-Wall, and how you can release it.

To find a Heart-Wall, you simply ask. Unless you actually *ask* the person's subconscious mind if they have a Heart-Wall, it will not be revealed.

The Heart-Wall is made of trapped emotions, but the subconscious mind no longer categorizes them as such. These emotions are now part of a wall and are inaccessible until you ask if there is a Heart-Wall. You have to get the mindbody to admit that there is a wall, before you can get to the trapped emotions that are creating it. Once you do that, the trapped emotions once again become recognizable to the subconscious mind as trapped emotions, and therefore, are vulnerable to being released. As you release them, one by one, the wall will come down.

It's really simple. Ask, "Do you have a Heart-Wall?" Then use the muscle test of your choice to get the body's response.

My experience is that about 80% of the general public will test positive for a Heart-Wall.

Use of the Word "Hidden"

When you ask, "Do you have a Heart-Wall?" and the answer is no, there might be another phenomenon at work. Quite often, the Heart-Wall will actually be hidden and will not show up unless you actually use the word "hidden" in your question or statement. The whole purpose of the Heart-Wall is to protect one's heart, or in other words, to *hide* the heart from those who might do it emotional harm. It seems that sometimes the Heart-Wall gets a bit *too* hidden to readily detect, but if you expressly use the word "hidden" when you ask, it will show up.

To check for this possibility, simply add the word "hidden" to your question or statement. For example, you could ask, "Do you have a *Hidden* Heart-Wall?" If they have one, and it's hidden, it will be revealed.

It's important to remember this tip. I can't tell you how often I've had to use the word "hidden" to find Heart-Walls that would otherwise not have been detectable.

A *hidden* Heart-Wall is not a different kind of Heart-Wall. It's simply a Heart-Wall that is a bit more difficult to find.

Once the body has opened up to you, to let you know that a hidden Heart-Wall is there, you can proceed without having to use the word hidden anymore, because it's no longer hidden.

Is it Ready to Be Released?

Once you have determined that a Heart-Wall is present, ask "Can we release an emotion from the Heart-Wall now?" The Heart-Wall is there for a reason, and while ultimately the effects of having a Heart-Wall are negative to the health and well-being of the individual, some people are in situations where they simply are not ready or willing to give up the protection of the Heart-Wall for now, and you need to respect that.

If a Heart-Wall is present, but you get a negative response about removing it, your subject may want to meditate on why the subconscious mind is giving that answer. Is it unsafe, or are they already processing some other things that are taxing the mindbody? At any rate, it is important to listen to their subconscious. It knows what is best for them.

If you get a yes answer to your question, you then simply follow the same process outlined in chapter six and follow it. For your convenience, there is a flowchart on page 278 that is specifically for releasing Heart-Walls.

The Emotion Code works the same way to release trapped emotions whether they are part of a Heart-Wall or not. When you ask, "Can we release an emotion from the Heart-Wall now?" and you get a positive answer, the mindbody has a particular emotion in mind that it is willing to release.

You don't get to choose which emotion will be released first; the subconscious mind of the subject will do that.

As soon as you receive a yes answer to this question, the trapped emotion has already been chosen. All you need to do now is determine which emotion it is on the chart, in order to bring it to conscious awareness. Identify it, determine any other information that the subconscious wants the conscious mind to know about it, and then release it.

Time to Process May be Needed

As I've explained previously, sometimes you will be able to release all the trapped emotions that are making up a Heart-Wall one after another, in one concentrated effort. At other times, the body will allow you to release a limited number of trapped emotions before needing to take time out to process what has been released, requiring from a few hours to a day or more before you can release another one.

After verifying the release of a trapped emotion from the Heart-Wall, you simply return to your original question and ask, "Can we release an emotion from the Heart-Wall now?" If the answer is yes, and if you have the time, keep going.

If the answer is no, you may want to check to see if perhaps the Heart-Wall is gone, by asking again, if they have a Heart-Wall. If they still have one, ask when you can release the next emotion – later today, in an hour, tomorrow, etc.

Determining the Heart-Wall Material

Remember that the subconscious mind is very logical. Since it is patently illogical to have a "wall" made of nothing, the subconscious mind will always choose a material for the Heart-Wall to be made of.

You don't really *need* to know what substance the subconscious mind chose to build the Heart-Wall out of in order to release it. Ultimately, all Heart-Walls are made of the energy of trapped emotions, and releasing these trapped emotions is what really matters.

On the other hand, determining the material that has been chosen is interesting because of the symbolism that is often revealed. There is no right or wrong way to ask what material has been used, but I usually start by asking if the material is wood. If it isn't wood, I ask if it is a material harder or softer than wood. If it is harder than wood, I may ask if it is made from metal, etc. You can narrow it down pretty quickly using the process of deduction, and you'll get some great practice using muscle testing.

If you have determined what material the Heart-Wall is made of, you might then want to ask how thick the Heart-Wall is. They can range in thickness from paper-thin to *many* miles! All I can tell you is that this is what we have found in testing. Our subconscious minds are not limited like our conscious minds are, and can have quite an imagination! Yet I believe that the subconscious mind takes it all quite seriously, and really does believe that there is a wall there, made of whatever material has been chosen.

Heart-Wall Metaphors

An older couple came to see me. The husband was very grouchy, and was dismissive and gruff with his wife. She seemed to be a very gentle soul. They both had Heart-Walls. His was made of solid steel, cold and hard, miles thick. Hers was many thousands of layers of curtain material, providing a nice cushion against his toxic personality.

A gay man had a Heart-Wall made of solid diamond, which is the hardest known naturally occurring material. Incidentally, his subconscious would not allow me to release this wall.

I've seen Heart-Walls made of flowers, quilts, blankets, earth, stones, vegetation, leather, glass, all kinds of metals such as steel, titanium, and iron, as well as various construction materials such as logs, concrete blocks, bricks, and so on.

Quite often there will be a noticeable relevance between the personality of an individual and their Heart-Wall material. I treated a young child once who had a Heart-Wall made of yellow plastic, just like her little yellow plastic toys.

Sometimes Heart-Walls will have a door or a window. Often the door will be locked, and nobody has the key but the owner.

While often a Heart-Wall is spherical, they can be box shaped, or any other shape you can imagine. Sometimes they have sharp edges or projections on their surface to keep people out.

One young man couldn't seem to form close attachments with women, although he was very handsome, had everything else going for him, and had many opportunities.

I found that his Heart-Wall was made of a one-way mirror, which allowed him to see out, but no one else to see in.

I once treated a child whose most common expression was "I can't!" I found and released his Heart-Wall. It was made from a single piece of paper. On it were the words, "I can't!" His parents commented that after his Heart-Wall was released, he no longer felt that he couldn't do things, and was happier and more positive. He also stopped whining and saying "I can't!"

Anne Horne's Story

A woman named Anne Horne wrote from Seattle to tell me of a remarkable near-death experience she had, in which she saw people in the future, helping others remove their Heart-Walls. Here, in her own words, is her story, or see the video at this link:

healerslibrary.com/news/anne-hornes-near-death-experience/

Dear Dr. Nelson-

I originally came into contact with your work when a practitioner here in Seattle named Marguerite used your techniques to balance my body. At the end of the session, Marguerite turned around and just as an afterthought said, "Oh, let's see if you have a Heart-Wall..."

"What is a Heart-Wall?" I said. "I don't understand."

And she said, "That's okay. You don't have to know what it is. I'll just test you for it."

So she did, and I didn't have one.

Then she said, "Let's test you for a hidden Heart-Wall."

"All right," I said. "But what is it?"

"That's okay," she said, smiling. "You don't have to understand."

She checked me for a hidden Heart-Wall, but I didn't have one of those either. Then she explained how emotions can put up a wall between yourself and others around your heart. When she found a Heart-Wall, she would run a magnet down a person's back to release those emotions and open their hearts.

I couldn't believe what I was hearing. It was like an electric bolt went through me. Suddenly, an event that had happened to me twenty-five years ago made sense. It was the realization of a very significant event that I'd experienced when I was 23 years old.

When I was 23, I died. It was a violent death. I had one of those near-death experiences that 10 million other people have also experienced. But when I was 23, nobody talked about this stuff. I'd never heard of seeing a tunnel or white light or anything like that.

It was a very important experience for me. I left my body and had a life review. I was a young thing and hadn't done anything particularly exciting or big. But I was going back, home, and on my way, there was a light, a tunnel. I felt like I was being pulled by my heart toward a wonderful place. In that moment, I was encompassed by all this innate intelligence and tremendous love. And I just wanted to go home. It was fantastic.

I found myself facing this man who was standing in front of me — we were not on the ground, we were just floating — and he said, "It's not your time."

I said, "But I want to go home."

He turned away from me and I could see him conferring with someone else, but I didn't know what they were saying. Then he turned around and said, "I'm sorry. It's not your time." But apparently, he did get permission to show me something about my life.

And suddenly, I realized where we were, because we looked down, and there was the earth. We were way out somewhere in space. And I could see the earth below us. We were looking at the Americas, specifically the West Coast of North America. We were looking at the Northwest area, Colorado, Texas, and down through California.

Now, I'm from Virginia and I died in North Carolina. At 23 years old, I had never even left the state. I was very young.

I could see many people in groups, sometimes large groups of 20 or 30, and sometimes just a few people together. They were in groups doing a specific training that was very unusual. There would be two or three people together, with one person lying on a table, or standing up, and another person who was rolling something down the other person's back.

I knew this was in my future, that I was one of these people. I could feel the sense of urgency that they were feeling. It was like a numbers game; we had to treat as many people as possible. We were really in a rush, really hurrying. It was very, very, very vital. I couldn't quite understand what was going on, but I noticed we were dressed in white.

"Are we nurses?" I asked him.

And he said "No, you're not nurses."

I said, "Well, what are we doing?"

"You're opening people's hearts," he said. "Not in a physical way. You're removing all blocks from their hearts so that they can give love and receive love from here."

At that moment, the people doing this work became consciously aware of each another. It wasn't something planned, it wasn't some kind of harmonic convergence, or anything else. It just happened. We became conscious of each other. And at that moment, the meaning of this work became clear to me.

Suddenly a flood of energy was sent to the earth from where I was, above the earth. It looked like a white bolt of energy that came in through our open hearts in the back and went out through the front of our hearts into the world. We were there opening people's hearts so that they could be anchors for this divine energy to come into this world.

Within three seconds, the world was completely transformed by this energy. This light went into every crack and crevice, everywhere, and there was no darkness in this world, ever again.

The next thing that happened was, the doctors resuscitated me and I was brought back to life. But it was OK because, once I got back, I pretty much thought that I had a mission from God. And I thought "Oh, my life is going to be so great!"

Well, my life has been a living hell! I have tried to have all kinds of trainings, looking for something that matched my experience on the other side, thinking, "Well, where is it? If this is my mission, when am I going to find out how to get started?"

I worked for the Edgar Cayce Foundation for Research and Enlightenment. I studied Quantum Physics for 25 years. I took courses in Physics of the Mind. I became certified as a Neurolinguistic Programming trainer and in hypnosis. I'm a graduate of the HeartMath Institute. I'm a trained counselor in chemical dependency, timeline therapy, and core transformation therapy. All the while, I've been doing my best to help improve people's lives, but searching for the connection between the work I was doing and what I'd seen.

I don't know if you've heard of the theory of the 100 monkeys. It's about reaching critical mass. There was an island of monkeys. Scientists came in and taught one monkey to wash his sweet potatoes. After 100 of them learned how to do it, all the monkeys on the island knew how to do it. Scientists thought that was pretty amazing. But that was only part of it. They soon realized that as soon as these 100 monkeys knew how to do it, the other monkeys automatically knew how to do it too. But not just the monkeys on that island. The monkeys on the islands all around that island began to wash their sweet potatoes, too!

It is like Dr. Nelson says, quantum physics has shown us that information travels instantly. If people's hearts are opened, we can reach critical mass.

During my near-death experience, I said to the man who met me, "But there are only thousands of us."

And he replied, "Millions will hear, but only thousands will remember."

And we only need thousands. Thank you for giving me a way to fulfill my mission. - Anne Horne

Counting the Cost

The price we pay for having Heart-Walls is incalculable. How many people have led disconnected and lonely lives due to the walls around their hearts? How many people have not experienced the joy of finding love in their lives? How many wives and children have been abused?

Heart-Walls can lead to depression, divorce, and abuse. The patterns of abuse that are created can pass from generation to generation, causing all manner of pain and destructive behavior.

The result of Heart-Walls on a larger scale leads to misunderstanding, prejudice, hatred and brutality. On a global scale, Heart-Walls lead to ethnic cleansing, nation against nation, terrorism, and war.

There is altogether too much of isolation and violence, too much of sorrow and pain in this world. When I walk down the street, I see so many people with tight, clenched jaws like Paula had or boys with angry, resentful expressions, acting out their pain and frustration any way they can. The news is filled every night with one story after another about people whose hearts must be barricaded behind strong walls for them to do the things they do.

Widespread depression is another common side effect of Heart-Walls and trapped emotions. In the

United States alone, it is estimated that between 13 and 14 million people suffer from depression. It is the leading cause of disability in American women. Nearly 15 percent of those women will ultimately commit suicide. Among children and young adults – between 10 and 24 years old – suicide is the third leading cause of death. By releasing trapped emotions and removing Heart-Walls, we have seen cases of severe depression eliminated once and for all. We have seen marriages saved, abuse stopped, and lives turned around. We've seen beautiful, loving relationships begin. We've seen kids make better choices. We've seen peace restored.

I am so grateful to be able to share what I have learned about trapped emotions and Heart-Walls, and to be able to bring this information to light. There is no doubt in my mind that it comes from above, and is meant to bless many lives in these times that are so trying in so many ways. I feel so blessed to have been led to discover a method that has such a powerfully transformative effect on people's lives. It's an exciting thing to be a part of.

If you have a Heart-Wall, can you see how important it is for you to clear that wall away? Can you see the importance of helping your own children and your own family? Can you see how transformational it would be if we could do the same thing for the whole world? Imagine how this world will change when we can open enough people's hearts to create a critical mass. As in Anne's near-death experience, that critical mass, perhaps only thousands of us, will be enough to help transform this planet forever. Those whose hearts are open will be the anchors for that divine energy that will transform and heal the world.

Imagine.

I wish I had the power to reach more people with the message of this book. If you'd like to share what you are reading with someone else — a close friend, for example — you can have this chapter emailed to them. Just go to:

HealersLibrary.com/freechapter

On the next two pages you will find a flow chart for releasing Heart-Walls, as well as the Chart of Emotions. I have placed them side-by-side so you can refer to them more easily when you are using the Emotion Code.

If you'd like to download a fully printable copy of the two following pages, simply visit my web site at:

HealersLibrary.com/flowcharts

Emotion Code Heart-Wall Flowchart

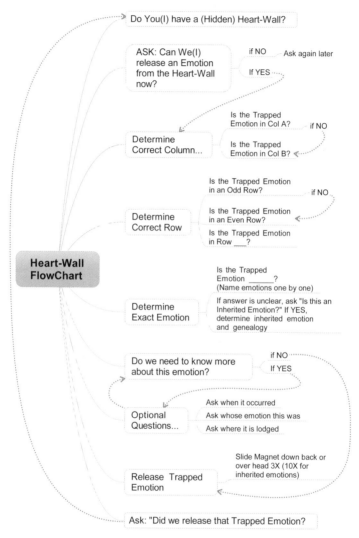

Follow the Heart-Wall flowchart above and the Chart of Emotions at the right to release Heart-Walls.

The Emotion Code™ Chart

	Column A	Column B
Row 1 Heart or Small Intestine	Abandonment Betrayal Forlorn Lost Love Unreceived	Effort Unreceived Heartache Insecurity Overjoy Vulnerability
Row 2 Spleen or Stomach	Anxiety Despair Disgust Nervousness Worry	Failure Helplessness Hopelessness Lack of Control Low Self-Esteem
Row 3 Lung or Colon	Crying Discouragement Rejection Sadness Sorrow	Confusion Defensiveness Grief Self-Abuse Stubborness
Row 4 Liver or Gall Bladder	Anger Bitterness Guilt Hatred Resentment	Depression Frustration Indecisiveness Panic Taken for Granted
Row 5 Kidneys or Bladder	Blaming Dread Fear Horror Peeved	Conflict Creative Insecurity Terror Unsupported Wishy Washy
Row 6 Glands & Sexual Organs	Humiliation Jealousy Longing Lust Overwhelm	Pride Shame Shock Unworthy Worthless

OFTEN THE HANDS WILL SOLVE A MYSTERY
THAT THE INTELLECT HAS STRUGGLED WITH IN VAIN.

- CARL JUNG

8

SURROGATES, PROXIES AND DISTANCE HEALING

Imagine being able to release trapped emotions on a loved one who is thousands of miles away. Imagine being able to tap into the subconscious mind of someone who is in a coma or unconscious and needs your help. Imagine being able to test your pet for trapped emotions and improve his behavior. All this and more is possible through two expanded forms of muscle testing that I refer to as surrogate and proxy testing.

Surrogate and proxy testing are probably the most useful adjuncts to muscle testing that have ever been discovered. I have taught many people to use these methods, and they have been able to use the Emotion

Code in what would otherwise have been impossible circumstances.

Although I have used surrogate and proxy testing for many years, I am continually impressed by how well they work. These forms of testing give you the ability to test otherwise untestable people, as well as to perform true distance healing.

I believe that we are living in an era when all the knowledge of past ages is coming back to the earth, and that the Emotion Code may once have formed part of that body of knowledge.

As we continue to refine our understanding of how the world works, we have made incredible advances in many areas. Things that would have been inconceivable in the past are commonplace to us today.

Just over a century ago, if you wanted to capture a likeness of someone, you had to draw or paint it. To create a full-color rendering usually took lots of paint supplies and many hours of effort. Now all you need is a tiny digital camera and a split second to press the shutter. Going to visit a relative 100 miles away used to be a week-long activity. Now, you can easily get there and back in half a day.

The task at hand is always made simpler when you have the right tools. Surrogate and proxy testing are powerful tools that can be used to effectively release trapped emotions regardless of whether that person is right in front of you or thousands of miles away.

Gifts from Above

I look on surrogate and proxy testing as gifts from above, gifts that allow us to get the job done even under trying circumstances.

For example, suppose you have a young child with an anger problem and suspect that a trapped emotion is involved. How do you muscle test a young child?

Suppose your husband who is overseas in the military is grieving over the loss of a comrade. How can you help him at such a distance?

Your dog becomes lethargic after one of your children goes away to college. You suspect there may be a trapped emotion involved, but how can you be sure? Your pet may understand a lot of what you say, but will they know what it means to "resist" when you do a muscle test? If so, please call me!

Surrogate and proxy testing allow you to use someone else as a substitute for the person (or animal) you're trying to test. Surrogate testing is used to test a person who is physically present, while proxy testing allows you to find and release trapped emotions from a person who is not present, and who may indeed be literally *anywhere* in the world.

Surrogate Testing

The following analogy will help you to understand how surrogate testing works.

Many small farms and ranches in America have low-voltage electrified cattle fences around their grazing areas. When a cow brushes up against the wire in an electrified fence, it receives a slight shock. These fences have proven to be simple, but effective at keeping cattle safely within their confines.

Not long after the first electric cattle fence was installed, farm boys made an interesting discovery. If one boy took hold of the fence, it was a shocking experience. The mild jolt of electricity pouring through his body was intense, but not life-threatening. If the boy holding onto the fence grabbed hold of another boy, suddenly that boy would experience the shocking discomfort, and the boy touching the wire would feel... nothing. He would merely be acting as the transmitter of the electricity, like an extension cord.

It didn't take long for this discovery to make its way around the farming communities. Just about anyone who grew up on a farm with an electric fence will tell you that they have tried this. I have spoken to people who remember being on the end of a long chain of people, and being continually shocked until they could get a hold of someone else to be on the end. It works.

Surrogate testing works on a similar principle. You can think of the subject who is actually being tested as the "live wire." They are the one with the electrical current you are trying to tap into. Because surrogate testing is always used on someone who is present, the surrogate simply touches the subject to make the connection. Then the testing is performed on the *surrogate*, rather than the subject.

Surrogate testing is the answer in any situation where a person is present physically, but is not testable.

Reasons that a person may be untestable might include the following:

1 Age, such as testing an infant, a small child or an elderly person.

2 Physical limitation such as injury, illness, pain, weakness, dehydration or neck misalignment.

3 Loss of consciousness such as sleep or being in comatose state.

4 Inability to reason due to mental retardation or if you are helping an animal.

Suppose you would like to test an infant. Anyone who is testable themselves, can act as the surrogate for the infant. In the case of a child, the surrogate could be the child's mother or father or anyone that the child is comfortable with. Of course, if someone other than a parent is testing a child, they should be sure to obtain permission from the child's parents before attempting to help them.

Anyone who is testable can act as surrogate for anyone else.

I've come to regard surrogate testing as an indispensable adjunct to muscle testing.

If you are getting an inconsistent response while testing someone, my recommendation is to put a surrogate in between, and perform the testing on the surrogate. The answers will be the same, and you will often find that using a surrogate will make it easier to detect the answers you are seeking.

You'll find that certain people are somewhat easier to muscle test than others. For example, my wife Jean is very easy to test, and since we work together, I often use her as a surrogate.

How to Do Surrogate Testing

The first step in doing surrogate testing is to make sure that the surrogate himself, is testable. Do this as we have previously discussed, by simply having the surrogate make a yes or no, true or false statement followed by a muscle test. Once you have a testable surrogate, proceed. Follow these steps:

1 To make the connection, the surrogate simply touches or holds hands with the subject.

2 Have the subject say their name in the form of a statement, "My name is ____." Muscle test the surrogate, who should test strong.

3 Next, have the subject make an incongruent statement by saying, "My name is_____," using any name that is not their own.

4 Muscle test the surrogate. The surrogate should test weak at this point. If not, repeat step three until they do. Once the surrogate tests weak when the subject makes an incongruent statement, the connection has been made and testing may proceed.

Within a few seconds after their initial physical contact, the surrogate and the subject will be connected and testing will be possible. Once this connection is made,

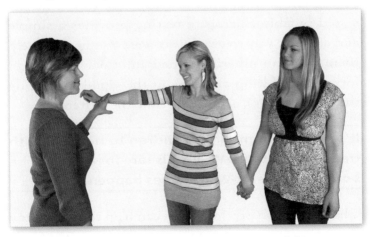

Tester　　　　　*Surrogate*　　　　　*Subject*

you will ask questions of the subject or have the subject make the appropriate statements, but the muscle you're testing belongs to the surrogate, not the subject.

Go through the questions described in the previous chapters to identify and locate any trapped emotions. Any change in energy that occurs in the subject will immediately flow through to the surrogate and become apparent through testing. To release a trapped emotion, pass the magnet down the back of the subject, if possible. If for some reason this is not possible, passing the magnet down the back of the surrogate will also work, provided they are still connected energetically.

The connection with surrogate testing is easy to break. The surrogate simply stops touching the subject.

Surrogate Testing Children

Young children are not usually able to be muscle tested reliably. Surrogate testing provides a simple and efficient way to get the answers you need to help them. We can inherit trapped emotions, or we can form them during our time in the womb or during the birth process, and at any time thereafter.

It's not uncommon for children to be born with trapped emotions. While it is rare for a child to be born with a Heart-Wall, it does happen.

Children are so precious! You can help them in many cases, simply by using a surrogate. The Emotion Code works the same way for children as it does for adults. Children that have stressful and difficult lives are certain to have trapped emotions, but any child can have trapped emotions, no matter how much love they receive or how favorable their home environment may be.

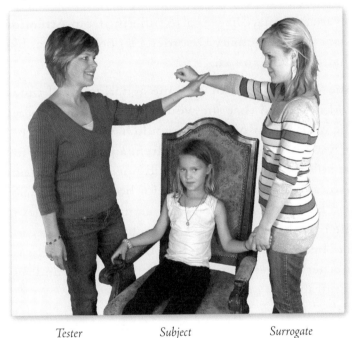

Tester   Subject   Surrogate

On the following pages is a dramatic story about how removing trapped emotions helped a very disadvantaged little girl in a very big way.

Julie's Story

Julie was a "crack baby." At one day old she was placed into the custody of a foster family who hoped to adopt her. Her problems were certainly not over with. When I first saw her at age two and a half, she had been diagnosed with Cerebral Palsy, Mental Retardation, and severe Asthma. She was also suffering from Attention Deficit Hyperactivity Disorder. Her behavior was like that of a wild animal.

She was in a state of extreme agitation at all times, and it seemed that she would have literally "climbed the walls" of my office if she could have. She could not play with toys or other children, and she could not sit still for a second. She could not speak at all. She had tantrums that would last for hours at a time. She had been hospitalized for her asthma seven times in the month before she was brought to our office, and had been on machines to help her breathe. Her foster mother was very patient with her, which I found very admirable.

By testing Julie through a surrogate, I was able to determine that she had a Heart-Wall, as well as other imbalances.

Here are the trapped emotions that were forming her Heart-Wall, which we were able to release, one trapped emotion per visit over a month's time.

Inherited Love Unreceived from Birth Mother

"Love unreceived" is a fairly common emotion which occurs when someone feels unloved or when their love for another is rejected. Julie's mother was suffering from a trapped emotion of love unreceived herself, and passed this on to Julie at the moment of conception.

As a society our natural tendency is to judge people like Julie's birth mother because of their addictions. We see the outward behavior and the poor choices that people like her make, and we tend to look down on them. But what we do not see is the invisible; the hurt, the sorrow and the grief that make up their own trapped emotions, their own Heart-Walls. Julie's mother had such a burden.

Inherited Hatred from Her Birth Father

We may never know what Julie's birth father had been through in his life that created hatred for him. Julie never met her birth father, but she was definitely affected by his trapped emotion of hatred. When trapped emotional energies pass from generation to generation, they interfere with how we would otherwise live. Emotions drive us to make the choices that we make. Emotions cause us to treat others the way that we treat them. Is it possible that trapped emotions that are inherited and passed from one generation to the next are partially to blame for generational abuse and dysfunction?

Grief and Anger from Her Birth Mother

Both grief and anger had become trapped during the first trimester of Julie's time in the womb. These two emotions were her birth-mother's response to being pregnant and had become trapped in Julie. These were the answers I received as I surrogate-tested Julie.

Grief, Disheartedness and Sorrow, Third Trimester

It is not unusual for a child to develop trapped emotions from the deep feelings that their mother is experiencing while she is carrying them. I found trapped emotions of grief, disheartedness and sorrow, all emotions that her mother was feeling during the third trimester. Trapped emotions are most commonly produced in the third trimester, but can be created at any time during pregnancy.

Hopelessness From Her Mother at Birth

Julie's mother was apparently feeling the emotion of hopelessness while she was in labor. Julie was still in her mother's body at this time, and within her mother's energy field. As her mother's body vibrated at the frequency of hopelessness, Julie began to resonate at that same frequency, and she was born with this trapped emotion.

Unworthy and Self-Abuse at Age One

The emotions of unworthy and self-abuse were created by Julie herself, because she had so much trapped emotional baggage compounded by toxicity from her mother's drug abuse. Her foster mother told me that when she was around this age she used to bang her head against floors and walls.

The Results

After Julie's third treatment she slept all night, and her breathing was no longer audible. By her fourth treatment her asthma symptoms were gone.

Shortly after her asthma symptoms disappeared, Julie's foster mother received a visit from her social worker. The social worker spent nearly two hours chatting with Julie's foster mother and filling out adoption paperwork. During this entire time, Julie sat on the floor and played quietly with her toys, something that she had never been able to do before. The amazed social worker asked, "What kind of medication do you *have* her on?" Betty replied, "Well, she is off all her medication now." Betty tells the story here in her own words.

We got Julie when she was a day old; she was a drug-exposed baby, and we planned on adopting her. She was sick, and in and out of the hospital at least 3 or 4 times a month with severe asthma, and was on a machine to help her breath, on prednisone and 2 or 3 other asthma medicines. She had cerebral palsy, and her behavior was just terrible.

We found Dr. Nelson for my mother, who was not doing well. And after seeing how far along she came, we decided to bring Julie to him. She has seen Dr. Nelson for 13 treatments, and when we came she was in the hospital 7 times in December, and she was on a machine. It's been 3 weeks since she has had any asthma medicine or the asthma machine or anything. She is doing really well. She is walking much better, and her bad behavior is almost gone.

She is talking now. When we started bringing her in, her speech was not there. She's talking, counting, and she is doing very, very well. We are very pleased and very happy with the results so far. She is just a different child. It was to the point that we didn't know if we were going to make it through a day with her or not between the asthma and her fit-throwing; she could have fits that would last for 2 and a half hours. Now she may get irritated but no fits, she might cry a little bit, but that's about it. We feel very happy and we feel very good! - Betty R.

Gratifying Results

Julie continued to improve, and before long, Julie's doctors informed Betty that they were withdrawing their diagnoses of cerebral palsy and mental retardation.

Her erratic and uncontrollable behavior were gone, and Julie was like a new little girl.

Our experience is that many behavioral and health issues that children have can be greatly improved or alleviated when the Emotion Code is employed.

In Julie's case, her health and mental development were greatly impacted as well. I can't express how gratifying it can be to free little children from the grip of trapped negative energies that have the potential to ravage their young lives.

Surrogate Testing Animals

Surrogate testing is the perfect solution for animals. Many animals could probably be tested directly— if they could understand how to participate in the test! But it's much more effective to enlist a surrogate on their behalf.

Let's say you want to test your horse. Simply ask the surrogate to touch the horse. Then direct your questions to the horse and test the surrogate to get the responses.

When I test animals, I always talk to the animal as if it were a human being. The animal may not understand the words, but they do seem to connect with the emotional intention that our thoughts convey. Believe me, animals understand what we're trying to do for them. Their ability to understand human intention may even exceed our own at times.

Surrogate testing works with cats, dogs and all kinds of animals. There are so many remarkable stories about using the Emotion Code on animals that I've devoted the next chapter to the topic.

Testing People Who are Unconscious

Surrogate testing also makes it possible to test someone who is unconscious, or even in a coma. Even if the person is unresponsive or unable to make verbal contact, their subconscious mind is still at work; it never sleeps. An unconscious person's bodily functions are still working. They are still breathing. Their heart is still beating. Their subconscious mind is still alert to the environment and working to keep things on track. When you ask the mind-body a question, the subconscious mind will know the answer, but if the person is unconscious, they will not be able to actively participate in the test. So testing through a surrogate is the perfect solution.

Muscle testing should never be used in an emergency situation, when CPR would be a more appropriate response.

A few years ago my father suffered a massive brain aneurysm and fell into a coma. I was deeply concerned and eager to help him in any way I could. When Jean and I went to the hospital to see him, we found it impossible to get close enough to work on him directly, due to all the tubes and wires that surrounded him.

I asked Jean to act as surrogate for my father. Even though he was in a coma, we were immediately able to tap into his subconscious mind and determine the things that we could do to help him the most, in addition to all that was already being done by the hospital staff. It was an unforgettable experience that made me grateful indeed, for the gift of surrogate testing.

Getting Permission

Just remember that you always need to obtain permission before you work on anyone, whether you are working on them directly, using surrogate testing or proxy testing. Here are some common-sense guidelines on who to obtain permission from in different scenarios.

Subject to be Tested	Obtain Permission From
Conscious Adult	Subject
Unconscious Adult	Subject's Closest Adult Relative
Minor	Minor's Parent or Guardian
Pet	Pet's Owner

Surrogate testing is such a useful tool that I have found it indispensable in reaching the full potential of this work. It makes it simple and easy to work on pets, infants, small children, the unconscious, and those who are either too weak or in too much pain to be tested.

Proxy Testing

When someone has been given authority to act for someone else, we commonly refer to the authorized person as a *proxy*. A proxy is someone who acts as a substitute. In proxy testing, the proxy temporarily "becomes" the person being tested. By voluntarily putting themselves into the position of standing in for someone else, a proxy can be tested as if they were the subject of the testing, allowing their body to be used to benefit the subject.

Proxy testing is most useful when you want to help someone who is not present or who is inaccessible for some reason. When you release trapped emotions from someone at a distance, it is literally a form of *remote* or *distance* healing. Although remote healing has not been incorporated into Western Medicine, it has been practiced both anciently and in modern times by those who practice The Silva Method, Qigong, GungFu, Reiki and other respected techniques.

Healing Allison in Japan

I once worked with a number of ballerinas from a local dance school near my practice. Allison, one of the dancers that I had been treating, went to Japan to dance with a group from Disneyland. Late one night, I got a phone call from Allison's worried mother. "Doctor

Nelson, we have a big problem," she said. "Allison has hurt her hip and can't dance. She is supposed to be in a big show tomorrow. Is there anything you can do?"

I told her I'd like to speak to Allison, so she gave me the number of her hotel in Japan. When I reached her, Allison described the problem with her hip and said it had started bothering her that day for no apparent reason, and that she was having difficulty walking. Dancing the next day was out of the question.

Having gotten permission from Allison's mother and from Allison to test her, I asked Jean to act as proxy.

Although Allison was literally on the other side of the earth, we had no problem making the connection.

We chose to call Allison on the phone in this situation to get her input, but it's important to note that proxy testing can be done without having the subject on the telephone while you are testing them. The energetic connection between the proxy and the subject is sufficient.

Distance is no barrier to energy. Energy is truly everywhere, and fills the world, and indeed fills the immensity of space.

There is as much energy in the air between objects as there is in the objects themselves. Since energy is continuous and everywhere-present, working on Allison presented no difficulty.

We discovered that Allison had two trapped emotions lodged in the tissues of her hip. The trapped emotions had to do with loneliness and grief over her trip to Japan.

"Do you feel that you don't want to be in Japan?" I asked Allison on the phone.

She grudgingly admitted it was true. "It's exciting to be here and all," she said, "but I'm very homesick. I miss my mom and my friends. I just really don't want to be here, and I wish I could go home."

By running a magnet down Jean's back, we released the two trapped emotions from Allison.

Even though Allison was half-a-world away in Japan, the results were instantaneous.

Before we hung up the phone with Allison, her hip pain was entirely gone. She went on stage the next day and danced without any problem.

Dorene's Remote Experience

A patient named Dorene wanted to share this story about how remote healing was just as effective for her as being there in person.

I have seen Dr. Nelson intermittently over the last 10 years or so for various problems. I had been suffering for several days with the symptoms of a hiatal hernia, including heartburn and pain. I was really miserable, and I wasn't getting anything done.

My husband, Rick and I were sitting in our family room when Rick decided to make a phone call to Dr. Nelson to see if there was anything that he could do to help me. He found through testing that my symptoms were being caused by a trapped emotion and he treated it. I can honestly say that the relief was instantaneous as we were sitting there and the symptoms completely left me before the phone conversation was over. I highly recommend that people be open to this type of treatment. There are wonderful discoveries available to us today through remote treatments by those who are knowledgeable.
- Dorene N.

How to Do Proxy Testing

Let's talk about the actual steps involved in doing a proxy test.

Above all else, you must obtain permission from the subject who is going to be tested. It's an invasion of privacy and is unethical to test someone without their permission.

Let's say that Ryan Jones would like to be tested and treated. He has given his permission to you and your friend, Susan to do so by proxy, since he is out of town. Susan has volunteered to act as proxy for Ryan, so you will be doing the testing on Susan.

1 As in any other type of muscle testing, you must make sure that the person who will be acting as proxy is testable, so perform a baseline test on the proxy first to make sure.

2 To establish an energetic connection between Susan and Ryan, have Susan make the statement, "My name is Ryan Jones." Now perform a muscle test. This statement will most likely elicit a weak muscle response at first. But the connection will occur if you persist a bit.

3 Simply have the proxy repeat this statement, (in this example, "My name is Ryan Jones") a few more times, each time followed by a muscle test. The clearer your intention to connect Ryan and Susan, the faster it will happen. Generally within a few attempts, the energetic connection will be made, and the muscle test will suddenly become strong.

To continue with this particular example, Susan will now test strong when she says, "My name is Ryan Jones." If Susan makes the statement "My name is Susan" she will test weak temporarily. Susan is now acting on behalf of Ryan. At this point, everything that is tested on Susan as the proxy, is actually being tested on Ryan, however far away he may be.

It's important to understand that when this energetic connection is made between the proxy and the subject, the connection is very real.

In some way that we do not understand, the needs of the proxy are entirely set aside temporarily in order to aid the subject.

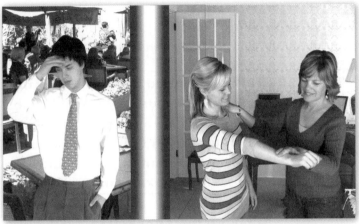

Subject   *Proxy*   *Tester*

Any question that you ask the proxy, you are now asking the subject. Any trapped emotion that you find by testing the proxy, you are actually finding in the body of the subject.

Until the connection is broken, anything that you want to test on the subject, you will simply test on the proxy; the answers will be the same. In this same way, any correction that you want to make on the subject, or any trapped emotion that you want to release on the subject, you will simply perform on the proxy.

As you can imagine, this is a very useful tool. It allows you to not only find out what trapped emotions are stuck inside the body of a remote person, but to release those emotions from afar — and often, relieve their symptoms immediately.

After the connection is made, you can use the Emotion Code the same way it has been presented previously. Ask questions and identify any trapped emotions in the subject, by testing the proxy.

When you identify a trapped emotion by testing the proxy, you can release it just as you would if the subject were there with you. Simply use a magnet on the proxy. Remember that energy knows no barriers of distance. Your intention to heal and your belief that it can be done make it so.

Breaking the Connection

Once you have completed this process, it is very important to "break the connection" between the proxy and the person being helped. If the connection is not broken, the proxy may actually begin to eventually experience the emotional state of the person they were acting as proxy for.

On one occasion, I had been using the Emotion Code to help a woman who lived in Cleveland. Her sister had been a patient of mine for some time at my clinic in California, and would act as proxy for her sister on occasion.

I once made the mistake of not breaking the connection between the two of them at the end of a session. The next day my patient came back to the office and said, "Something is wrong. I feel like I'm turning into my sister. I'm feeling her emotions, I think. It's weird. Could I still be connected to her?" I immediately realized my mistake, broke the connection, and she felt like herself again.

When you are finished, thank the person who has acted as proxy. To break the connection, simply have the proxy state their own name and muscle test them until they test strong.

For example, if the proxy's own name is Susan, have her say, "My name is Susan." If she tests weak, she is still connected to the subject. In that case simply ask her to repeat the statement with her own name in it until she tests strong. That's how you know the connection is broken. It's just that simple.

Something Special

I feel that there is something truly sacred and special about healing using a proxy. The way that the subconscious mind of the proxy subordinates the self in favor of the subject is amazing. The knowledge of how to do this, as well as how to make the connection at any distance, is hard-wired into us all.

I am always thrilled when I work with someone long distance by proxy and the subject finds an immediate improvement or release of symptoms. I hope you will give both surrogate and proxy testing a try. Anyone can do it, including you.

Though I am confident that you can learn to do proxy testing with practice, I find that some of my readers are interested in having our help.

If you are interested in having a certified practitioner help you you remotely using proxy testing, please visit either or both of these two links:

Staff Practitioners: HealersLibrary.com/services

Global Practitioners: HealersLibrary.com/practitioners

We have a growing number of practitioners around the world who spend their time releasing trapped emotions from their clients by proxy, which means they can work with you as well, no matter where you are on the planet. For more information about this topic, see page 369.

Surrogate testing is particularly useful when it comes to helping your pets. In the next chapter, you will hear a lot more about how amazing the Emotion Code can be when used on animals.

ANIMALS CAN COMMUNICATE
QUITE WELL, AND THEY DO.
AND GENERALLY SPEAKING,
THEY ARE IGNORED.

- ALICE WALKER

9

THE EMOTION CODE
AND ANIMALS

As any animal lover will tell you, animals have feelings, too. They may not be able to talk about them, but if you watch their behavior and get to know them, you will soon be able to recognize their subtle changes of emotion. Even without words, animals express their emotions clearly. When emotionally upsetting events occur, animals can suffer from trapped emotions just as people can.

A Horse is a Horse, of Course...

My first experience treating trapped emotions in animals occurred somewhat by accident. One day, I received a telephone call from a patient named Linda, a trainer from San Juan Capistrano. She had come to me a year before with a rather severe case of asthma that I'd helped her with, but this call was about something else entirely.

"I have kind of a strange request and I'm wondering if you can you help me," she said. "One of my horses, Ranger, is having a problem with frequent urination. I've had three veterinarians examine him, but none of them can find out what's wrong. As far as they can tell, he's perfectly healthy. But he's causing a terrible problem – not just for me, but the adjacent stall owners and horses as well. I know that you occasionally work on animals, and I'd really appreciate it if you could come to the stables and see what you can do."

When Linda had come to my office for her own treatments we'd talked about our shared love of horses. I had grown up around horses in Montana and never missed an opportunity to ride. Linda had shown me photos of four or five beautiful horses she kept in her stables, but I'd never been to the stables to see them.

The next day, Jean and I made the trip down to Linda's stables. We walked into a large, rectangular building with a peaked roof that covered about forty horses' stalls in two rows. As we arrived at Ranger's stall, we could see immediately why Linda was so concerned about him. Unlike all the other neat, clean stalls we had seen in the building, this horse's stall was a soggy mess, as he was having a urination problem.

Linda brought Ranger outside so we could work on him on dry ground. Jean volunteered to act as surrogate, and put one hand on the horse, holding her other arm out for me to muscle test.

We determined that there was something causing an imbalance in Ranger's kidneys, but after testing him for a few minutes, I was at a loss as to what the source of the imbalance might be.

"Why don't you test to see if there's a trapped emotion?" Jean said.

I laughed out loud. "Test a horse for trapped emotions? That's really funny…" I was born and raised in Montana, and had two different horses of my own while I was growing up. While I loved my horses and took good care of them, like most people, I never imagined that they might suffer from trapped emotions.

Jean looked at me calmly and repeated, "Just test and see." Jean is very intuitive, and she was probably sensing the truth about what was going on with Ranger.

So I asked out loud, "Is this imbalance due to a trapped emotion?" and pressed down on Jean's arm. The answer was "Yes."

As I went through the chart of emotions, we were surprised to find that the trapped emotion was "conflict." By a process of elimination, we determined that Ranger felt conflicted in his relationship with another horse. Linda was able to confirm that a new horse had been brought into the stables in the past few months. Ranger and this new horse were at odds from the first day they met and occasionally had to be separated to prevent them from injuring one another. They had moved the new horse further away from Ranger's stall, but the two horses still came into contact with each other almost daily, if only in passing.

Further testing showed that this trapped emotion had become lodged in the right kidney, and was indeed the underlying cause of Ranger's kidney imbalance.

Once we had verified the trapped emotion, I released it by rolling a magnet down Ranger's back. When I retested Ranger through Jean it was apparent that the trapped emotion had been released.

From that moment on, Ranger began to recover. When I talked to Linda on the phone a few days later, she told me that his stall was dry for the first time in months. The problem never recurred.

Although I rarely worked on animals, as my practice consisted almost entirely of people, this experience opened a whole new dimension for me, and it can for you, too.

Working on Animals

Releasing trapped emotions from an animal is essentially no different than releasing trapped emotions from a human being. You will use the same Chart of

Emotions that you are already familiar with. The only psychological hurdle you might have to overcome is that you will be speaking directly to the animal, or rather to the subconscious mind of the animal, instead of the subconscious mind of a person. Everything else is pretty much the same.

1 Since you will be using a surrogate to test the animal, perform a baseline test on the surrogate to make sure they are testable.

2 The surrogate will place one hand on the animal and hold their other arm outstretched, to be used for muscle testing. The tester will then make sure the animal and the surrogate are connected by asking the animal a simple question. For example, if you're working on a horse and the horse's name is "Buck", you might ask the animal "Is your name Buck?"

3 Muscle test the surrogate, and when the surrogate tests strong when congruent questions are directed to the animal, and weak when incongruent questions are directed to the animal, the connection is made.

Once the energetic connection is established, you can test the surrogate for answers as if you were testing a human being. For all practical purposes, there is no difference.

Your first experience testing an animal may really surprise you. To suddenly open a line of communication with an animal is a fascinating experience that is oftentimes quite moving.

Twiggs Gets Dognapped

A little Lhasa Apso named Twiggs is a perfect example. His owners, Brett and Cathy, told me his story when they brought him in.

A few months before, they had all been taking a walk together in the foothills near San Juan Capistrano. Twiggs, who was very inquisitive and loved to go exploring, had trotted off down the trail about 50 or 60 feet in front of them. Suddenly, there was a rustling of leaves and a coyote emerged from the brush along the trail. A heartbeat later, the coyote was running away with Twiggs in his jaws. Brett and Cathy barely had time to move before he was gone. They chased the coyote into the trees, but there was nothing they could do.

Going back home, broken hearted, they resigned themselves to the loss of their dog. They were still grieving four days later, when Twiggs showed up on their doorstep. He stood there quivering, his hair all matted and bloody, glad to be home. They rushed him to the animal hospital, where the vet stitched up his wounds, gave him antibiotics, and saved his life.

"It was like a miracle," Cathy said, stroking Twiggs, as she held him snugly in her arms. "We were so relieved!"

"So what seems to be the problem?" I asked.

"He's just not the same dog any more," Brett explained. "He never barks or chases anything. He seems to have lost his interest in life."

"And he shakes all the time," Cathy said, holding Twiggs up so I could see how much he was trembling.

"The vet says it might be neurological damage," Brett added. "He said there's nothing he can do. It's probably permanent."

Cathy set Twiggs down on the table, so I could examine him. I checked for misalignments in the spine. I found a few, as I had expected, and adjusted them.

"The thing is," Cathy said, "We're wondering if we should put him down…."

"His quality of life just isn't very good any more," Brett said. "He never barks or runs around like he used to. We have to carry him everywhere. His curiosity is gone. He just seems like he's suffering all the time."

We all looked at Twiggs, sitting on the adjusting table, shivering, with a miserable, frightened look in his eyes.

I could only imagine the terror he must have experienced when he was attacked and carried off, and decided it was likely he was suffering from a trapped emotion. After getting permission from Brett and Cathy, I explained surrogate testing and asked one of them to act as surrogate for Twiggs.

When I asked if he had a trapped emotion, the answer was "Yes." I assumed that the emotion would be fear or terror. As I narrowed the list of emotions, what turned up was surprising. The emotion that filled this little dog's heart and soul at the time it was being carried off by the coyote wasn't terror, or anything like that. It was sadness.

As he was being carried off in the jaws of the coyote, all Twiggs could think about was that he was never going to see Brett and Cathy again, and the thought overwhelmed him with sadness.

Once we identified the trapped emotion, I quickly released it with a magnet and the treatment was over.

When I set Twiggs down on the floor, he took off like a speeding bullet! He ran down the hall and into the waiting room. When he had first come into that waiting room, in Cathy's arms, he'd been shivering so hard, he hadn't seemed to notice any of the people there. Now, he greeted each patient with several nice, healthy barks. Then he rushed down the hall and stuck his head into every room, barking at least once, before he finally ended up in front of Brett and Cathy, happily wagging his tail.

It was an amazing, instantaneous transformation. We were all astonished and touched by this miraculous healing. According to his owners, Twiggs stopped shaking from that moment and his charming, inquisitive personality returned.

The great thing about testing animals for trapped emotions is that what you see is what you get. Animals don't pretend they're feeling better just to make you happy. Often the effect is immediate, and quite profound.

Twiggs seemed to know that we were trying to help him. And when he suddenly felt better, the change was obvious to everyone!

Brandy's Naughty Behavior

We dropped in to visit with some friends at their home one evening, when I was "greeted" by their dog Brandy in a very enthusiastic, but rather obscene way.

"I'm so sorry!" Skip said. "Every time we have guests over, he rushes up and starts humping their leg! It's really embarrassing, and there's nothing we can do to get him to stop, so we finally have resorted to locking him outside when we have company. We didn't realize you were going to stop by, otherwise he would have been locked out in the backyard."

As we sat with them our conversation quickly turned to other topics, but from where I was sitting I could see poor Brandy on the other side of the sliding glass door, looking forlorn.

Changing the subject of our conversation back to Brandy, I told them that a trapped emotion could be the cause of his odd behavior. They hadn't heard of anything like this before, but they trusted me and were willing to let me check Brandy.

It didn't take long to determine that my hunch was right. Brandy's trapped emotion was grief, and here is how it happened.

The family had recently purchased a cabin in the mountains. At first, they'd taken Brandy with them in the backseat, but he couldn't endure the long drive. He kept getting carsick and throwing up in the car. Soon they started leaving him behind. Brandy would get all excited, watching them pack up their gear, and then they'd drive away without him. Brandy was distraught, and didn't understand why he was left behind when he was so excited to go and be with them.

That's when the trouble started. They had never had any trouble with Brandy before, but suddenly Brandy was different, and when a visitor would come to the house, Brandy would rush them and hump their leg, to everyone's disgust. Apparently, he couldn't express his grief any other way.

Once we cleared the trapped emotion, that behavior totally stopped. The family still didn't take Brandy to the cabin, but at least he got to be in the house full-time again.

Boofy the Paranoid Cat

The unique thing about this story is not so much what happened to her cat, but how a young woman discovered her own gift and found a new direction in her life.

After my friend, Cyrena, and I finished Dr. Nelson's two-day seminar on trapped emotions, we were eager to try out our new knowledge. When we got back to my house, we both spotted my cat asleep on the couch and thought "Aha! Our first victim!"

Boofy was a stray cat that adopted our family when he was about one-year old. We had cared for him well and had even given him a collar with a bell, so he wouldn't get lost again. We tried for a month to find his owners, but when we couldn't, we decided to keep him because he was so well-behaved.

Although he was always friendly with us, Boofy had a terrible fear of strangers. Instead of rubbing up against their legs, looking for attention, like most cats do, Boofy seemed to see all strangers as a threat. If someone Boofy didn't know came into the room, he would bolt and run.

Using myself as a surrogate, I tested Boofy for trapped emotions. As we suspected, the trapped emotion was fear. Once we cleared the trapped emotion by running the Magboy down his back, Boofy rolled over to have us scratch his stomach, but nothing else particularly happened.

But a few days later, when a visitor came over, we noticed that he didn't run. In fact, when any new person came into the room, Boofy now acted like any other cat, sometimes going up to them for petting and attention.

Thanks to Dr. Nelson's training, I've found that I enjoy working with animals. I've even discovered that I have a special ability for working with them. Using self-testing, I can identify trapped emotions quickly and clear them. I have my own pet therapy business now, and have seen for myself the remarkable changes that come to animals using the Emotion Code.

- Katrina B., Washington

Abandoned Puppies

I received another touching letter from Katrina, who has become very proficient at using the Emotion Code with animals.

Last year, I received a phone call from one of my friends asking if they could borrow our boat. They had been at a private park by the Stillaguamish River when they thought they heard whimpering puppies. After looking around, they saw the puppies by the cliff across the river, stranded on a small sandbar. My friend was afraid that the next rainstorm would raise the river and drown the puppies, so she needed my boat to rescue them.

My brother Ben and I took our canoe to the park and rescued the puppies. One was already dead, but we took the other four home with us. They were beautiful black puppies with white markings, a mixed breed of pit bull and German shepherd.

One of them would not stop shivering, even when I wrapped it up in a blanket and held it next to me. I knew it wasn't cold, it was in shock. But I got out my emotion chart and started testing for trapped emotions, using myself as the surrogate. The puppy's primary trapped emotions were terror, shock, fear, betrayal and abandonment.

As I worked with the puppy, asking questions about what had happened and testing myself for the answers, I learned that the puppies had been deliberately abandoned and left there to drown. It's easy to understand how upsetting that would be! I carefully cleared all of the trapped emotions from the puppy and confirmed that they were gone.

After less than a half-hour of work, the puppy had stopped shivering and calmed down. Even though I was happy to keep holding him snugly in the blanket, he wanted to get up and play.

Knowing the trauma these puppies had been through, I cleared the trapped emotions from the other puppies, too. I wanted to be sure to give them a better start with the families that would adopt them when we took them to the animal shelter. The pound had no problem finding them good homes.

- *Katrina B.*

A Horse's Sorrow

After I'd worked on Ranger, word started getting around about my unusual approach to treating animals. An owner asked if I would come to look at her horse, Valiant, who was having difficulty with his gait, or the specific pattern of his leg movements.

Valiant was an elegant horse used in dressage, a particular kind of horse training in which the horse learns to follow very specific movements by the rider. With an abnormal gait, it's impossible for a horse to work, so Valiant's training had ground to a halt. A veterinarian had seen the horse, but could find nothing physically wrong, so Karla, the horse's owner, turned to me for help.

My arrival at the stables caused a bit of a stir. The owners, horse trainers and stable hands were curious to see this new technique that purportedly freed horses of their emotional baggage. A small crowd gathered around the stall as I worked. I asked for a volunteer to act as a surrogate and a rider named Melissa volunteered.

As I tested Valiant through Melissa, I soon found the reason for his gait problem. There was a trapped emotion that was imbalancing his hind-quarters.

Further testing revealed that the trapped emotion was sorrow.

"Is it sorrow about another horse?" I asked. Melissa's arm went weak, which meant "No."

"Is it sorrow about a human being?" Her arm went weak again. "No."

"Is it sorrow about a dog?" "No."

"About a cat?" "No."

Knowing it would help to know the nature of the sorrow, but running out of possibilities, I kept at it. Seeing a squirrel nearby, I asked, "Is it sorrow about a squirrel?" "No."

"Is it sorrow about a bird?" At this point, Melissa's arm tested strong, indicating a "Yes."

A horse feeling sorrow about a bird? This somehow struck me as being quite funny, and I started to laugh, along with everyone else. This was really unexpected.

Suddenly, Karla, the horse's owner, spoke up. "Wait a minute. I think I know what this is about."

I could see from the look on her face that she was serious. "Last week," she said, "a baby bird fell out of its nest onto the road, right in front of Valiant's stall. The baby bird struggled for its life for a time, but it ended up dying."

"Is this sorrow about the baby bird that died?" I asked Valiant through Melissa. The answer was "Yes."

Valiant must have seen the whole thing. As this baby bird struggled helplessly for its life and eventually died, Valiant was overwhelmed with sorrow, and a trapped emotion was formed, which was imbalancing his hind-quarters and affecting his gait.

Running a magnet down his back, I released the trapped emotion. Karla led him out of the stables and walked him. Lo and behold, Valiant's gait problem was suddenly gone, along with his trapped emotion of sorrow about a little baby bird.

Amazing Horse Stories

Our children were taking riding lessons at a local equestrian park and we ended up treating the owner's horses for trapped emotions. The owner tells the story here.

I have been involved with horse training and riding since I was fourteen years old. I now own and operate an equestrian facility. I regularly compete in National Reining Horse Association events around the country with my horses.

I met Dr. Nelson and his wife, Jean a year or so ago, and have been privileged to have the two of them work on some of my horses, with amazing results, and I would like to share with you what I have seen.

All my horses are quarter horses, and are considered working cattle horses.

One of my favorite horses is Newt. He is now 14 years old, and has been retired for 5 years, which is very unusual for a horse, but Newt has some problems. About 10 years ago, Newt slept on an anthill, and was bitten repeatedly by ants in a large area of skin over his left hind-quarter. Within a few days, all the hair fell out of that area, and he never really recovered from it. Although the hair grew back, I quit showing him about 6 or 7 years ago, as he just couldn't perform any more, and it was obvious to me that he was in pain. His energy level was very low, and it seemed that he was suddenly old before his time. Over the last five years he has been totally retired, but I have been taking him out about twice a year to work him just a bit, just to give him something to do.

Over the years I have had vets look at him, chiropractors, and even tried shock therapy, but nothing worked at all. Newt is a very valuable horse. Both of his grandparents were from DocBarr twice, from both mother and father. DocBarr is a very famous quarter horse. His mother's lineage is in the top 5 reining and cow-horses in the country.

As Dr. Nelson and Jean worked on Newt, they told me that he was suffering from trapped emotions. Specifically, he had lack of control and nervousness from around age 2. This dated back to before I had him, when he had been worked too hard and too aggressively by his former owner/trainer. They said he had some sort of disconnection going on in the left hindquarter, dating back to the ant bites as well.

Since Dr. Nelson and his wife worked on him, (he had a total of one treatment that lasted about 30 minutes) Newt is like a new horse. In fact, it's like he has suddenly gone back to where he was when he was a four-year-old. I can now use him to rope cattle, which puts a lot of strain on the horse's back, with no problem. I can rein him and put him through all his paces, and he performs at the top of his game. It's amazing to me how he acts now. He is full of energy, and wants to play all the time. After being retired and unable to do much of anything at all for many years, Newt is brand-new.

Another horse of mine I call Buck. He is probably the best horse I have, and is a beautiful little buckskin quarter horse. I got him three months ago. From the very beginning, he was suffering from a severe lack of energy and trust, and had no desire to do anything. He didn't want to work. I happen to know how he was trained, and it was way too aggressive, to put it kindly. My observation *is that you can get a horse to perform with that kind of harsh training for about a year, and then you are all done, because the horse finally says, "You can hurt me all you want, and I just don't care anymore. I'm done."*

Well, Buck had reached that point, and he was done. He hated his life, hated his job, and hated people, because they had mistreated him so much. Dr. Nelson and his wife checked him out, and found trapped emotions of hatred at age 3 (he felt that the trainer hated him), depression at age 3, and other emotions of overwhelmed, panic, and feeling taken for granted.

Since then, Buck has changed in a big way. His cadence has changed, he is much smoother to ride, and feels much more relaxed, which is how he should feel to me when I ride him. In addition, he is no longer afraid of people, and much less guarded. He is now a normal horse in all those aspects, he loves to work now, and is full of energy. It's really amazing. He is like a new horse.

Last month, I took Buck to the NHRA show, where he took 3rd out of 30 head in the stallion class event, and 3rd in the trainer horse event. I am happy to say that he beat his old trainer's best by five points at this show. Training by instilling fear might work for a while, but trust lasts forever.

I'm not sure how Dr. Nelson's method works, but I am absolutely convinced that trapped emotions are real. It is truly amazing to see this process done and to see the results that are obtained. Without Dr. Nelson knowing anything about a horse's history, the emotions and things that come up are exactly right on.

I have seen this method work, and I can see and feel the results in my horses. When I try to describe it to people they say it sounds like Voodoo. All I know is, it works, and that's all I care about.

- Boyd Roundy, Utah

More Amazing Horse Stories

My name is Debbie Spitzenpfeil. I am an FEI level Dressage Trainer and Clinician, and I have trained in Germany with Olympic trainers. After having a training barn in San Juan Capistrano, California for 17 years with 23 horses from Training Level to Intermediare II, I am now semi-retired in Oregon with my Holsteiner Stallion, Revelation. I teach Dressage Clinics in Oregon, Colorado, and California as well as judging shows in these states.

I attended the first seminar on magnetic healing that Dr. Nelson held, in San Diego, California, in July of 1998. I have used his methods of clearing trapped emotions and have found them to be invaluable in working with horses, as well as people, and I have many amazing stories that I could share, but here are a couple of great ones.

One horse that was in training with me for several years would go lame several times a year. We had three different vets look at him, x-rays, chiropractic, and acupuncture done but nothing seemed to work during these times. It was very frustrating since we were competing with him and never knew just when this mysterious lameness would occur. When I learned the Emotion Code through being a patient of Dr. Nelson's for 10 years, as well as going to his seminars, I began to use energetic balancing on the horses I had in training with me.

Highlander would go lame in his right hock area. I began to clear his emotional baggage. He had a Heart-Wall that was 29 stalls thick. I was able to eliminate all of the Heart-Walls through clearing. He had abandonment issues, anger and resentment at his owner, and major grief. I was able to trace this back to when he was 5 years old and was being trailered. He had fallen down in the trailer. The owner never stopped to help him and he had to lie that way the entire trip. I asked the owner if this had indeed happened and she ashamedly admitted that it had. She simply did not know what to do, so drove with him in the trailer until she got to the show grounds. Highlander knew that she knew, and he resented her for it. He also felt abandoned by her.

After I was able to clear everything, he went from being totally lame in the hock to being completely sound within 10 minutes. He remained sound for the next 3 years while I had him in training. Only two times did I have to clear him again, and that was when he saw horses that didn't want to load into a trailer and I think he recalled his grief. But still he stayed sound and went on to win several Championships.

Another horse I was training in a clinic came in lame. I had never taught him before. I asked his owner if I could muscle test him to see if this was a physical lameness or an emotional one. It was an emotional lameness. I was able to clear his grief issues over the loss of another horse that had to be put down in his barn. He was mourning the horse and short-circuited in many organs as well as his heart. It took me about 10 minutes to clear him, after which he immediately trotted off sound. He continued to be sound for many more Clinics until he was sold to another home.

I have used the Emotion Code on horses I plan to purchase to see if they have emotional short circuits and if they are indeed trainable. It has helped me enormously in choosing good horses. I am always muscle testing my horses to do check-ups on their health status. I think they are physically healthier and happier because of Dr. Nelson's methods.

- Debbie Spitzenpfeil, Oregon

Conclusion

We populate this earth along with the animals, and many times we end up in the position of being their caretakers in a very personal way. They are our companions and our friends. We sometimes come to love them as if they were another member of our family, and this is as it should be.

Like our family, it falls to us to make sure the animals in our care are fed and sheltered, and to do our best to keep them safe and healthy.

Keep an eye on the animals in your care. If something unsettling happens – like the baby bird dying right in front of Valiant – think about how your animal might feel. When an animal develops symptoms of any kind, whether they are physical or behavioral, they may reflect a trapped emotion. You now have the tools to help them on your own.

Don't be afraid to try. Just let your heart be full of love for the animal, have a prayer in your heart, have a clear intention to help them, believe that you can do it, and you will be successful.

PART IV

A BRIGHTER FUTURE

I AM NOT AFRAID OF TOMORROW,
FOR I HAVE SEEN YESTERDAY AND I LOVE TODAY.

- WILLIAM ALLEN WHITE

10

LIFE WITHOUT TRAPPED EMOTIONS

To live a life completely free of trapped emotions would truly be a wonderful thing. It might be achievable, but from what I have observed, there is rarely a person that does not get a trapped emotion from time to time. It seems to be part of the human experience.

Life is a mixed bag, filled with blessings to be grateful for, difficulties to overcome, opportunities to explore, decisions to make, and grief and suffering at times. All of these things give us experience. They provide ways for us to exercise faith, gain knowledge and develop love. All of the human family is connected and everything that happens to one of us affects everyone to one degree or another. Through our experiences we have the opportunity to strengthen our connection by developing understanding and compassion for one another.

The way you decide to feel each day with all of the many things that you face will determine how life will flow for you.

Your attitude has tremendous bearing on what will present itself before you, on the opportunities that will come, and on what you will learn.

In reality, you attract much of what you see before you because of what you believe you can have in your life.

Your Focus Determines Reality

The choice is there each new day, to feel good or to feel bad about the things that are going on in your life. There are almost always both good and not-so-good things happening at any given time. What you choose to focus on is a big factor in the happiness equation.

Sometimes people put too much focus on the past. If you choose to focus your mind on a negative event from your past and re-experience those emotions, you can actually create a trapped emotion about that event, even long after it has happened.

One particular patient named Diane comes to mind in this regard. Diane's father had died 10 years previously, yet I found a trapped emotion of sorrow about his death that she had created 4 years after he died. While she had made it through his funeral without creating any trapped emotions, she had chosen to allow the negative emotion of sorrow to overcome her on the fourth anniversary of his death. At that time, she had made a conscious decision to re-experience her loss and sorrow, instead of thinking about the wonderful and positive things that her father represented to her. The result was a negative and potentially dangerous trapped emotion.

Stop for a moment and think about your own thoughts. During any given day of your life, do your thoughts tend to be more positive or more negative? Do you choose to dwell on favorable, positive things and decide to feel grateful, content and joyful or do you choose to dwell on negative emotions?

If you are in a troubled relationship, for example, there are almost always a number of good things that you *can* think of that you appreciate in your partner. Focusing on the good things about a relationship and giving your attention to its positive aspects can help to create gratitude and happiness for you. To do so may even open a way to create positive change, especially if it is your intention to build and preserve the relationship.

By contrast, whenever we place our focus on our problems and on the things that are going wrong in our lives, we end up creating more negativity. I saw a movie once where a wise teacher told his student,

"Remember, your focus determines your reality." How true that statement really is! You can see a glass as being half-full or half-empty, but seeing the glass as half-full is more empowering and will create a more positive reality for you.

The Law of Attraction

Feeling positive emotions about what you want will literally help you to create your dreams. When you visualize your life the way you want it to be and feel the way that it feels as if you already had your dream, you will eventually find opportunities to create the things that make you happy right in front of you.

Focusing on the things that you don't want and feeling negatively will either create or perpetuate those same negative problems in your life.

For example, if you spend your time thinking about how you can't seem to find love, the signal you are sending out to the universe is that you can't find love. As a result, you won't find it, or it will at least be more difficult to find.

We are constantly radiating our thoughts into the cosmos. I believe that these thoughts fill the immensity of space, and that they are not limited by the speed of light or any other limitation. Our thoughts are powerful, and what we think and feel is what we create.

Remember Proverbs 23:7, "As a man thinketh in his heart, so is he."

Creation is always happening. Every time an individual has a thought, or a prolonged, chronic way of thinking, they're in the creation process. Something is going to manifest out of those thoughts... And so you end up attracting to you the predominant thoughts that you're holding in your awareness, whether those thoughts are conscious or unconscious.

- Rev. Michael Beckwith[1]

You may already understand the importance of controlling your conscious thoughts, and keeping those conscious thoughts in a positive vein. But what about your subconscious thoughts?

Your subconscious mind can have a very great effect on the outcomes that you are trying to achieve in your life. Trapped emotions work their negative influence on you in large part through the mechanism of your subconscious mind. You may be trying your best to think positively and see the glass as half-full, while your subconscious trapped emotions are betraying you by constantly radiating their own particular negative thought-frequencies into the universe.

The more trapped emotions you have, the more negative thought-energy they are radiating, and the

---

1 *The Secret*, TS Productions, LLC. 2006.

more difficult it will be to attract what you really want.

The good news is that trapped emotions can be released. When you make a habit of using the Emotion Code regularly, you will be able to avoid the damage that occurs on a subconscious level of thinking and feeling because you will be changing your thought-frequencies.

When you free yourself of negative trapped emotions, you will find it easier to choose the positive emotions that will help you to attract what you really want in your life.

You Choose Your Emotions

Have you ever made a statement like, "My husband makes me so mad…" or "That made me so depressed…" or "That put me in such a bad mood"? Statements like these are very common. If you listen to yourself more closely you might catch yourself saying something similar. If you stop and think about statements like these, you will realize they're quite ridiculous. The fact is that nobody can *make* you feel any emotion that you don't *choose* to feel.

Things that happen *to* you do not really determine the emotions that you feel. While you may not have conscious control over all of the events that affect your life, you do have the ability to choose how you think, feel, and act. No matter what happens, you ultimately choose the emotions that you feel.

Many of us unwittingly become victim to our emotions at times. You may not believe that you are in control of how you feel. Negative emotions can emerge so quickly that it may appear as if there is no time to choose a different emotion than the natural reactive emotion that just seems to come out of nowhere. If you are late for an appointment, you may automatically feel anxious. If someone treats you rudely, you might automatically feel miffed. When you are insulted or abused, you may immediately feel resentful or angry in response.

If you are like most people, unacceptable things happen from time to time. Unless you take control of your emotions, you will simply react. When you allow yourself to react, your subconscious mind may offer up a negative emotion for you, based upon the emotions you have chosen in similar circumstances in your past.

While you may have always responded in a certain negative way to a given situation, your past negative responses do not have to be the same as your future responses. You have a choice every time you need to deal with or confront something negative. You can choose to react how you have always reacted or you can choose differently. The past does not have to equal the future.

The reality about emotions is that you *always* choose them. You always choose how you feel. Always. Becoming aware of this is in itself quite empowering. You are the author of your own emotional experiences.

You can choose whatever emotion you want in any situation you are faced with. It takes some practice, and it's not always easy, but it can be done.

The next time you find yourself filled with a negative emotion, stop and think about the process you went through to arrive at that feeling. It might seem like the emotion chose you, but you really did choose the emotion.

Making a conscious choice instead of allowing old subconscious patterns to run you is choosing to evolve and grow.

Using your new knowledge and awareness of trapped emotions will help you to be able to stop and think before letting an automatic response get the best of you.

The next time you are faced with a negative situation, don't simply react. Think! Ask yourself, "Which will serve me better, a negative emotion or a positive emotion?" My guess is that positivity will usually win. There are all kinds of great ways you can choose to feel. Here's a list of positive emotions that you can use the next time you want to choose positively.

Positive Emotions List

Acceptance	Delight	Hope
Ambitiousness	Diligence	Humility
Anticipation	Elation	Interested
Awe	Empathy	Joy
Benevolence	Excitement	Kindness
Calmness	Faith	Love
Charity	Forgiveness	Modesty
Comfort	Friendship	Passion
Contentment	Generosity	Patience
Confidence	Gladness	Peace
Courage	Gratitude	Satisfaction
Curiosity	Happiness	Surprise
Desire	Honor	Willingness

About Letting Go

In the book "Man's Search for Meaning" the importance of choosing your own emotions instead of allowing negativity to choose you is illustrated very well. Dr. Victor Frankl was a psychologist who was sent to a concentration camp by the Nazis during the Second World War. As a student of human behavior, Dr. Frankl naturally began to observe the people around him. People's reactions to their predicament and the horrors they observed around them varied widely. Dr. Frankl found that those people that chose the emotion of hopelessness, and who simply gave up did not survive for long.

To his surprise, Dr. Frankl found that in the midst of indescribable horror there were still those individuals that chose emotions of love and hope. He wrote:

"We who lived in concentration camps can remember the men who walked through the huts comforting others, giving away their last piece of bread. They may have been few in number, but they offer sufficient proof that everything can be taken from a man but one thing: the last of the human freedoms—to choose one's attitude in any given set of circumstances, to choose one's own way."

About Pride

When you hear the word pride, what do you think of? Pride in an accomplishment? Pride in a job well done? Perhaps you think of pride in your athletic team or pride in being the citizen of a certain country. While all of these kinds of pride are probably quite all right, there is another kind of pride that is insidious and damaging.

The kind of pride that hurts us is sometimes called false pride. It is when we put ourselves in a state of opposition to others or to God. It is when we feel hatred, jealousy, resentment, superiority, ill will, or anger toward another. False pride is selfish. It can be like a temper tantrum, when our way is the best and only way.

False pride is often very difficult to recognize in ourselves; it has been called "the great vice" because it is so common among people. One of the real problems with this kind of pride is that it makes you unwilling to forgive others. Instead, pride makes you want to hold on to the real or imagined hurts you have suffered, and leads you to all kinds of negative emotions such as anger, frustration and resentment. Eventually you may end up wanting revenge on those who may have wronged you.

When we pit our own will in resistance against others or against God or the Universe, we steal our own power. The source of all power is God; if we are working against Him we paralyze ourselves and stop our progress.

In reality, allowing false pride to persist in your life only thwarts your own progress and hurts you. Pride of this sort leads to the creation of trapped emotions, because it does not allow you to let go and forgive; it does not allow you to access a higher path that leads toward peace. Instead, pride leads down the dark road of negative feelings, usually beginning with a feeling of resentment.

Anger will never disappear so long as thoughts of resentment are cherished in the mind. Anger will disappear just as soon as thoughts of resentment are forgotten.

- *Buddha.*

About Forgiveness

It is so important to realize that letting go of old hurt feelings helps *you.* You may think that you are justified in holding on to hurt feelings because it punishes those that hurt you. In reality, holding on to negative emotions hurts *you*, not them. They may or may not be aware of how you feel, but the way *they* feel is entirely up to them. Just because you choose to suffer by holding onto the past doesn't mean they will suffer along with you.

They may have truly done something horrible. It may seem impossible to let it go. This is where you have power to do something meaningful that can be life changing, especially for you.

You can decide to forgive them, thus freeing yourself of all of the negativity associated with the problem.

I've always liked this quote by Lewis Smedes, "To forgive is to set a prisoner free and then discover that the prisoner was you." So why not set yourself free? Why create more negativity and more damage by feeding your hurt feelings year after year?

Have a mind to let things go. Forgive. Problems happen so often out of ignorance.

So much human suffering is because we don't know what we do to one another. If only we could understand that what we do to others, we do to ourselves.

If you've been mistreated, think of the example left for us by Jesus Christ, who said these words as he was being nailed to the cross, "Father, forgive them for they know not what they do." In his extremity, he chose the emotion of love and forgiveness, and we can, too.

A true-life example of the power of forgiveness made national news in 2005. Columnist Jay Evensen tells the story:

> How would you feel toward a teenager who decided to toss a 20-pound frozen turkey from a speeding car headlong into the windshield of the car you were driving? How would you feel after enduring six hours of surgery using metal plates and other hardware to piece your face together, and after learning you still face years of therapy before returning to normal—and that you ought to feel lucky you didn't die or suffer permanent brain damage?

> And how would you feel after learning that your assailant and his buddies had the turkey in the first place because they had stolen a credit card and gone on a senseless shopping spree, just for kicks? . . .

> This is the kind of hideous crime that propels politicians to office on promises of getting tough on crime. It's the kind of thing that prompts legislators to climb all over each other in a struggle to be the first to introduce a bill that would add enhanced penalties for the use of frozen fowl in the commission of a crime.

> The New York Times quoted the district attorney as saying this is the sort of crime for which victims

feel no punishment is harsh enough. 'Death doesn't even satisfy them,' he said.

Which is what makes what really happened so unusual. The victim, Victoria Ruvolo, a 44-year-old former manager of a collections agency, was more interested in salvaging the life of her 19-year-old assailant, Ryan Cushing, than in exacting any sort of revenge. She pestered prosecutors for information about him, his life, how he was raised, etc. Then she insisted on offering him a plea deal. Cushing could serve six months in the county jail and be on probation for 5 years if he pleaded guilty to second-degree assault.

Had he been convicted of first-degree assault—the charge most fitting for the crime—he could have served 25 years in prison, finally thrown back into society as a middle-aged man with no skills or prospects.

But this is only half the story. The rest of it, what happened the day this all played out in court, is the truly remarkable part.

According to an account in the New York Post, Cushing carefully and tentatively made his way to where Ruvolo sat in the courtroom and tearfully whispered an apology. 'I'm so sorry for what I did to you.'

Ruvolo then stood, and the victim and her assailant embraced, weeping. She stroked his head and patted

*his back as he sobbed, and witnesses, including a
Times reporter, heard her say, 'It's OK. I just want
you to make your life the best it can be.' According to
accounts, hardened prosecutors, and even reporters,
were choking back tears.*[2]

About Charity

The ability to forgive others arises from our own ability
to love. The purest form of love is unconditional love,
also known as *charity*.

One of the most well-known scriptures from the New
Testament is 1st Corinthians chapter 13, which reads
in part:

1 *Though I speak with the tongues of men and of angels, and have
not charity, I am become as sounding brass, or a tinkling cymbal.*

2 *And though I have the gift of prophecy, and understand all
mysteries, and all knowledge; and though I have all faith, so that I
could remove mountains, and have not charity, I am nothing.*

3 *And though I bestow all my goods to feed the poor, and though I
give my body to be burned, and have not charity, it profiteth me
nothing.*

4 *Charity suffereth long, and is kind; charity envieth not; charity
vaunteth not itself, is not puffed up,*

5 *Doth not behave itself unseemly, seeketh not her own, is not easily
provoked, thinketh no evil;*

6 *Rejoiceth not in iniquity, but rejoiceth in the truth;*

7 *Beareth all things, believeth all things, hopeth all things, endureth all
things.*

---

2 Jay Evensen, "Forgiveness Has Power to Change Future," *Deseret Morning
News*, 21 Aug 2005, p. AA3).

8 *Charity never faileth: but whether there be prophecies, they shall fail; whether there be tongues, they shall cease; whether there be knowledge, it shall vanish away.*

How can forgiving others and having charity help you to avoid getting trapped emotions?

Charity is love, pure and simple. Unconditional love for our fellow-beings. I believe it's really one of the most important reasons we are here on this earth; to learn to develop this kind of love.

When we feel this way toward others, our hearts resonate at the frequency of love, and we experience peace and harmony within.

This frequency doesn't allow room for any of the dark feelings that could create trapped emotions.

Charity helps us to get out of ourselves, to get beyond our own self-centeredness. It helps us to be more interested and understanding of the needs of others. It leads us to sacrifice of our time, service, and worldly goods to give to another in need. It helps us to become *givers* and grateful *receivers* rather than *takers*. It creates a bond, a kinship, a brotherhood between us. It gives value to us as individuals, and gives us wholeness and a sense of belonging.

Charity, this pure love, is a gift from God, and emanates from the heart. Since it is a gift from God, we can ask Him for this gift, and we should.

When our hearts are filled with charity, we are turned outward, not inward. We find joy in helping to create happiness for others. Our concern for the welfare of others becomes as great a concern as our own happiness. We therefore create our own happiness by making worthwhile contributions to others and to society. Our hearts enlarge in a spiritual sense, becoming more capable of giving and receiving love.

Mother Teresa is universally admired for her service to mankind. She was asked how she could continue day after day, visiting the dying, feeding them, touching them, wiping their brows and comforting them.

She said, "It's not hard, because in each one I see the face of Christ in one of His more distressing disguises."

When our hearts are full of charity, we are much less likely to develop trapped emotions. We are forgiving, patient, and kind.

Our tendency is to overlook the faults and weaknesses of others, rather than to judge them. A life full of charity is worth striving for and worth living. It is a life of positivity, a life that is high above the sea of negative emotions below.

About Integrity

When we live congruently with what we know to be right and true, we have integrity. Integrity is a virtue, an inner strength, an honesty with one's self. Integrity drives people to be their best selves.

Generally, the more integrity we have, the less likely it is that we will develop trapped emotions because the soul is not divided, but is whole. There is no tearing of the heart, no conflict within.

When a person chooses to live in integrity, he is at peace with his own heart and mind.

When he continues on this path, integrity grows, confidence strengthens and positivity increases. A person living this way has little room for negative emotions that might become trapped.

Life, by its very nature, is uncomfortably challenging at times. We must meet those challenges by growing and going through change, so those with integrity are not exempt from trapped emotions entirely.

Personal growth requires stretching, adjusting, accommodating the needs of others, refining ourselves, taking risks, making difficult decisions, and doing more than we thought we could.

Adversity, opposition, and challenge certainly do give us the opportunity to grow. We can choose to resist and resent those challenges or welcome them as blessings, and feel gratitude for the growth they will bring to us. Sometimes the experiences that are the hardest to face, benefit us the most.

When we go through times of opposition, we may need to check ourselves for trapped emotions that might result, to stay free from their negative effects.

The Refiner's Fire of Life

Life is a learning and purifying process. There's a story that illustrates this principle very well.

There was once a group of women studying the book of Malachi in the Old Testament. As they were studying chapter three, they came across verse three, which says: "He will sit as a refiner and purifier of silver." This verse puzzled the women, and they wondered what this statement meant about the character and nature of God. One of the women offered to find out about the process of refining silver and get back to the group at their next Bible study.

That week this woman called up a silversmith and made an appointment to watch him at work. She didn't mention anything about the reason for her interest beyond her curiosity about the process of refining silver. As she watched the silversmith, he held a piece of silver over the fire and let it heat up. He explained that in refining silver, one needed to hold the silver in the middle of the fire where the flames were hottest as to burn away all the impurities.

The woman thought about God holding us in such a hot spot — then she thought again about the verse, that he sits as a refiner and purifier of silver. She asked the silversmith if it was true that he had to sit there in front of the fire the whole time the silver was being refined.

The man answered "Yes", and explained that he not only had to sit there holding the silver, but he had to keep his eyes on the silver the entire time it was in the fire. If the silver was left even a moment too long in the flames, it would be damaged.

The woman was silent for a moment. Then she asked the silversmith, "How do you know when the silver is fully refined?"

He smiled at her and answered, "Oh, that's easy. When I see my image in it."

If today you are feeling the heat of this world's fire, just remember that God has His eyes on you.

- Unknown

If the trials of your life seem overwhelming to you, remember that God has a purpose for you and that you are loved.

God is refining you. He will know you are finished with this process when He can see his own image when he looks into your face; when you have become like him in your ability to give unconditional love.

I believe that each of us has a destiny to fulfill, and a mission to perform while we are sojourning on this earth. Trapped emotions can contribute to illness and can prevent us from living the life we could be living. It is a sacred calling to help those who are suffering, not only because of themselves, but also because the ripple effects of their life, lived fully, can spread out through time and space to eternity. Some of the greatest satisfactions in my life have come from teaching people, bringing out the healer in them and practicing the healing art myself. As I do these things, I experience the joy that comes from empowering others and helping them to be well and happy.

About Prayer

When I was a young man, I had a profound spiritual experience, in which I learned that God is real. I know that He lives and that He loves us all. We are His spirit children, brothers and sisters in a very literal sense.

Prayer has been an essential key for me in understanding who we as human beings really are, how our bodies really function, how to correct problems and how to heal. It has been my custom to ask a silent prayer for guidance before attempting to help anyone who has come to me for help. Many times I have received understanding and inspiration that was beyond my own. I am grateful for this help, and I give the credit to God for it.

I strongly encourage you to ask God for help in all areas of your life, and especially in your attempts to help others. He will be there for you. You have only to believe and be grateful that He is helping you.

In case you are not sure how to pray, or what format you might follow, I will share with you what has worked for me.

I start by simply addressing God, usually by saying, "Heavenly Father", as I believe He is my father.

I next thank Him for the opportunity I have to help the person I am trying to help.

Then, I ask Him for His help to do this, and for His insight and guidance.

Lastly, I close my prayer in the name of Jesus Christ, Amen. The word Amen simply means, "so be it."

God bless you on your journey to getting well yourself. I hope that you will help many others along your way. I know that you can.

Dr. Bradley Nelson

ABOUT THE AUTHOR

Dr. Bradley Nelson graduated with honors from Life Chiropractic College West, in San Lorenzo, California in 1988. He has lectured internationally on the natural healing of chronic illness, and was in private practice until 2004, successfully treating patients from across the US and Canada who were suffering from Chronic Fatigue Syndrome, Fibromyalgia and a wide variety of other chronic ailments. A holistic chiropractic physician and medical intuitive, Dr. Nelson is one of the world's foremost experts in the emerging fields of bioenergetic medicine and energy psychology.

Widely renowned as a speaker and a gifted teacher, he is now making his teachings available online at HealersLibrary.com, a membership site providing 24/7 access to Dr. Nelson's acclaimed Emotion Code Seminar instructional videos, webinars, television and radio interviews, books, certification materials and more.

Dr. Nelson is married and is the father of seven children. He lives with his family in Southern Utah.

HealersLibrary.com

My goal is to provide the knowledge that will help empower you to become a healer. I believe this is your birthright; to know how to help yourself and your loved ones to shed their emotional baggage and their heart-walls, that all might live up to their full potential.

I have created HealersLibrary.com for the express purpose of making these powerful natural healing techniques and supplements available to everyone. Stop by and see how easy it is to be a member of this online educational library where you can:

‣ Watch The Emotion Code Seminar online

‣ Access videos, books, CDs, tools and supplements

‣ Ask questions and interact with other students

‣ View our schedule of live & online events

‣ Order more copies of The Emotion Code

‣ Find out about how to become a Certified Practitioner

‣ Purchase remote sessions

‣ Watch live webinars on The Emotion Code

At Healerslibrary.com, you can watch the Emotion Code Seminar videos, connect with others, watch exclusive members-only training videos, and start taking advantage of all the site has to offer by visiting this link: HealersLibrary.com/subscribe

Seminars

I'd like your group or organization to be successful! Imagine what it would be like to have your entire team free of their Heart-Walls and other trapped emotions that are interfering with your success! We are available to teach the Emotion Code to your sales team, leadership and management on request. Just send an email to: Seminars@HealersLibrary.com

Interested in Teaching?

We are looking for people who are interested in helping us to teach The Emotion Code to the world. If you are interested in becoming one of our certified instructors, please visit this page: HealersLibrary.com/future-instructors

Healing Tools

I have found that trapped emotions can be released by using magnets of all types and strengths, as well as zero-point energy devices. Simply sliding your fingertips over the governing meridian will release a trapped emotion, since the body has it's own energy field. Nevertheless, there are healing tools available that not only work well with The Emotion Code, but are very beneficial in other ways as well, and as long you are using The Emotion Code to help people, you may want to consider the following tools:

Nikken Magnets

Personally, I prefer to use the magnets manufactured by the Japanese company, Nikken, Inc., because they are specifically designed for use on the body, and are very comfortable to use. The magnets that I use to release trapped emotions are designed to roll down the back, are easy to hold, and as they spin, they produce a larger magnetic field.

I still use them whenever I can. I have found numerous applications for them (for example, to reduce discomfort, where a refrigerator magnet would not have the same effect). I believe that the Nikken magnets are well worth the modest investment required.

Many years of clinical research in Japan has gone into the design and creation of Nikken's magnets, and they work very well. In fact, all the stories in this book that involve the use of magnets to release trapped emotions are referring to Nikken magnets.

The two specific magnets that I recommend for practicing The Emotion Code are both made by Nikken. They are the MagBoy, a small, hand-held magnet that can easily roll over the governing meridian, and the MagCreator, a larger, beautifully designed massage tool made with heavy-duty roller bearings, built to last. Either one of these is ideal.

If you'd like more information on any of the Nikken[1] products go to: HealersLibrary.com/nikken

---

1 The statements contained in this book do not express the views of Nikken and have not been approved by Nikken. Nikken does not market it's products for medical use and the products are not intended to treat, heal or cure any disease or disorder.

The Body Code

The Emotion Code is part of a larger body of work that I call the Body Code System. During my years in practice I developed a very simple, yet comprehensive method of addressing any and all imbalances that a person might have. This system worked extremely well for me, even with the most difficult cases. Using The Body Code, it is possible to tap into the subconscious mind to find and fix nearly any kind of imbalance, whatever it might be. I had always had a vague plan to teach this system to doctors at some undefined future day. A few years ago, however, I awoke one morning with the very clear instruction that I must take everything I had learned about healing and create a self-study course, so that this knowledge could be had by everyone, everywhere.

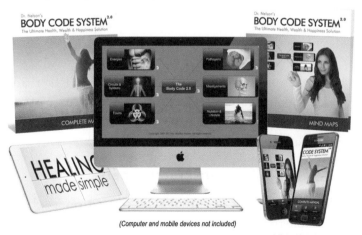

(Computer and mobile devices not included)

The Body Code System - A Comprehensive Self-Study Course

It took a year for me to create the Body Code System, but it is now available. I believe it is without doubt the most comprehensive self-study course on energy healing that has ever been devised, and consists of 18 DVDs, 2 manuals, an interactive mind-map for your computer, and more. For more information, please visit: BodyCodeHealing.com

Get Certified!

We offer certification in both The Emotion Code and The Body Code for individuals that are interested in helping others as a career.[2] Please note that certification in The Emotion Code is a prerequisite for becoming a certified Body Code practitioner. There is a growing need for certified practitioners worldwide, and you may be able to help us fill that need. For more information please visit this link: HealersLibrary.com/certification

Need Help?

If you are interested in having a Certified Practitioner release your trapped emotions and/or Heart-Wall by proxy or in person, we have a growing family of people who can help.

Staff Practitioners

We have a select group of staff practitioners that are available to work with you. You can make an immediate

---

2 The information contained in these materials is intended for personal use and not for the practice of any healing art, except where permitted by law. No representation contained in these materials is intended as medical advice and should not be used for diagnosis or medical treatment.

appointment online at a time that is convenient for you, and your appointment will take place over the telephone. The most popular appointment offered is the "Emotion Code/Body Code Session via Telephone" in which your Certified Body Code Practitioner will address as many imbalances as your body allows, including Trapped Emotions (usually 5-8 imbalances). This is usually a 20 minute appointment which is done by proxy, over the telephone. For more information or to make an appointment visit: HealersLibrary.com/services

Global Practitioner Map

At HealersLibrary.com we have a global list of Certified Emotion Code and Body Code Practitioners that will be happy to help you lose your emotional baggage and get your life back in balance. If you are looking for someone in your local area, our Global Practitioner Map makes it easy to find just the right person for you.[3] Simply browse the list and choose a practitioner at this link: HealersLibrary.com/practitioners

Facebook & Twitter

Please join us on Facebook at HealersLibrary.com/facebook

To follow The Emotion Code on Twitter, visit this link: http://twitter.com/#!/TheEmotionCode

To receive Twitter posts on your cell phone, text "follow TheEmotionCode" (leaving out the quotatation marks) to 40404 in the United States.

3 Please note that not all practitioners offer in-person sessions

Bulk Ordering/Book Customization

To contact the author or to request information regarding bulk rate book purchasing or book customization for your corporation or group, please contact: Orders@HealersLibrary.com or write to us at:

Wellness Unmasked Publishing
HealersLibrary.com
450 Hillside Drive Bldg A 225
Mesquite, NV 89027

Got a Question?

If you have a question about The Emotion Code, chances are it has already been asked and answered. Please visit our knowledgebase at: HealersLibrary.com/support where you can see the questions other have asked, as well as asking any question you may have that not yet been answered.

Important Addresses:

General Help: CustomerService@HealersLibrary.com

To contact Dr. Nelson regarding media appearances, please email: PR@HealersLibrary.com

INDEX